P9-DIW-611

Healthy Body / Healthy Home Melaleuca Guide

Dr. Richard Brouse
&
Julie Brouse-Conrad

Sixth Edition - Copyright 1996
Health Education Corporation

Copyright 1996 Health Education Corporation

6th Edition
(May 1996)

All rights reserved. No part of this book may be reproduced in any manner without permission in writing, except in case of brief quotations embodied in critical articles and reviews.

Health Education Corporation
8800 SE Sunnyside Road, Suite 111
Clackamas, OR 97015

(503) 243-1213
(800) 845-2025
FAX (503) 654-3056

NOTE

This book is intended to supply educational information to users of products containing oil of Melaleuca alternifolia. It should not be used as sales literature or for business promotion.

TABLE OF CONTENTS

INTRODUCTION

Since my first book, *Melaleuca: Nature's Antiseptic* was published in 1986, I have had thousands of cards, letters and phone conversations on my weekly Hot Line from users of this wonderful product. Many have requested that we add more complete descriptions of health conditions and their care. We are delighted to oblige. If you have used earlier editions of my book, you will notice that this edition has been expanded to include conditions that go beyond the skin because of increased interest in total natural health care. One thing is certain, health care reform is happening! People are taking control of their health as never before. Patients are asking the right questions, and health care providers are responding with *patient centered* information. Prevention, practiced at home, makes sense.

This 6th edition is no longer just a skin care guide. It is now a total health guide. With the addition of the *Vitality For Life Personal Health Risk Appraisal* and its associated products, a new awareness of health has emerged. In light of this breakthrough, we have been able to add our clinical observations for a greater number of health conditions of interest to our Melaleuca using patients and their friends. While the *Vitality for Life* program gives a wonderful introduction to major known factors that can influence your health, we have attempted to bridge the gap created between this wonderful risk appraisal program and the need for seeking a physician.

We have introduced, in this edition, the revolutionary *HEALTH TALK*, a 24 hour telephone health advisor. This program was developed ten years ago by our professional programming staff to give our patients easy access to health information any time of the day. It gives timely advice for common health concerns. It is as easy to operate as the Automatic Teller Machine, but with real voices. We encourage you to make use of it.

More articles and books are appearing on the subject of natural health care than ever before. Over one thousand scientific articles are published each week on studies that can help us with our health. New information is constantly available from even casual reading magazines. Journalists and lay health writers are compiling information from numerous sources to help educate an information-hungry public. However, most people are having difficulty sorting through all of this often conflicting information coming from many different sources. Some of this information is second hand or hearsay, being stated as *facts* and it is often used out of context. Almost anyone can write on a topic involving health these days having little experience and no training in the subject. The difference between this book and other books on the subject, is that this book is based on scientific research, as well as my 20 years of clinical experience with Melaleuca Oil. Consider the sources of your information.

I hope you will find that having this information at your fingertips gives you and your family greater control of your health. My purpose in writing this booklet is to empower people with greater awareness of proven natural health alternatives and thus prevent many self-imposed illnesses.

Drawing of Healthy Skin

MELALEUCA OIL AND HEALTHY SKIN

Healthy skin produces many different essential oils to maintain equilibrium with the environment. Each cell of the body has a double fatty envelope that makes up its' membrane. This is what separates the cell from its' environment. It is the character of this envelope to allow highly selected gases, nutrients, vitamins, minerals, hormones, and water into the cell while excreting wastes with a precision unique to life itself. When *Melaleuca alternifolia* oil is put in contact with healthy cells, only the Creator of both could describe the complex interactions which take place. Several things are known about plant oils and human skin. Incompatible ones such as oils of Poison Ivy activate a response to flush the substance away from the system. Essential oils are absorbed and mix delicately with the equilibrium and further the harmony of health. Bacteria have an electrical charge on their surface, much like the electric polarity of a battery. Friendly bacteria have a similar electrical charge to the skin cells they protect. Essential oils, such as found in *Melaleuca alternifolia* oil, encourage the growth of these friendly bacteria. Potentially dangerous bacteria have a lower electrical charge and are destroyed by these oils. Viruses do not carry any appreciable electrical charge and their protective lipid coats are dissolved by essential oils, allowing them to be chemically destroyed by the body's natural defenses. What do we understand about *Melaleuca alternifolia* oil and this symphony of life at the molecular level? Actually, not much more than what the native Australian people shared with Captain Cook - try it and see what its properties can do for you.

PERSONAL NOTES

MEDICINE CHEST AND PERSONAL CARE PRODUCTS

NOTE: Melaleuca medicine chest and personal care products are unique in their concept and design in that they all have the oil of *Melaleuca alternifolia* (composed of at least 48 naturally occurring oils) as a base. Because of their biologically active ingredients, like food, occasional sensitivity may occur. Persons who have known sensitivities to plants or foods should not be alarmed if some skin reaction occurs. For sensitive skin, apply smaller amounts, or less frequently than suggested, or dilute 1:1 with pure olive oil. The most highly refined form, *T40-C5*, has the lowest percentage of Cineol (an irritant to sensitive skin) which makes it more easily used over a broader range of conditions. Occasionally, sensitive skin is an indication of basic nutrient deficiencies. Take *The Vitality Pak* and *G'Day Melaleuca Tea* for several weeks and then retry the product. You may find that when your nutritional status improves, you are no longer sensitive to the product.

◆ *Antibacterial Liquid Soap*

A pleasant smelling disinfectant soap for skin, hair and wounds. In combination with *T36-C7* it is a must for camping trips and first aid kits. Caution - avoid eye contact.

◆ *At Last! Anti-Perspirant/Deodorant*

With the proven power of safe perspiration retarding ingredients, *At Last!* controls the cause of body odor. Bacteria cannot grow without the nutrient rich environment of perspiration.

◆ *Body Satin Lotion*

Skin lubrication is essential for proper moisture content. This product made with oil of *Melaleuca alternifolia* sets a standard for proper protection of easily damaged skin. This is an excellent lotion for massage and easily irritated skin.

◆ *Breath-Away*

This is a very effective mouthwash with its oil of *Melaleuca alternifolia* which promotes fresh breath and healthy gums. After normal brushing, make a 1:4 dilution of this concentrate with water and brush, gargle or swish.

◆ Defend Deodorant

This fresh herbal scent not only is pleasing to smell but offers confidence when in close contact with others. Preventing body odors by inhibiting bacterial growth naturally, is an added feature of this product.

◆ Dental Gel for Kids

Preventing cavities can begin early with this sugar free and abrasive free natural fruit product. Developing healthy habits early is easier when the experience is pleasant for children. They want to brush after every meal when the tooth brush can taste this good.

◆ Dental Tape with T36-C7

If you have ever had dental floss break while flossing your teeth, you will appreciate the tested double strength of the Dental Tape. The addition of *T36-C7* makes this a wonderful *"below-the-gum"* preventive product.

◆ Denti-Care Tooth Polish

A fine quality tooth polish which contains oil of Melaleuca alternifolia. This paste stimulates and disinfects gums and gingival crevices.

◆ Exfoliating Hydration Masque

As a deep cleanser this product containing oil of *Melaleuca alternifolia* disinfects and protects delicate skin.

◆ Gold Bar

Containing *T36-C7* in a natural glycerin base, this bar soap not only cleans and disinfects, but also preserves natural moisture in dry skin. This is the only bar soap that has these properties.

◆ Hand Creme

For hard working hands, this hand creme with oil of *Melaleuca alternifolia* gives maximum protection against cellular damage and promotes rapid healing of dry skin. This unique formulation moisturizes and penetrates to soothe, soften and protect your hands, feet, elbows and knees - anywhere that needs extra protection.

♦ Herbal Shampoo

Some people enjoy the fresh smell of nature's medicines on their hair. Combine *T36-C7* with the natural hair conditioning effect and here is a shampoo for maintaining healthy hair and scalp.

♦ Hot Shot Mouth & Throat Spray

A refreshing breath spray containing oil of *Melaleuca alternifolia*. After eating out or enjoying odiferous foods, this pleasant spray cleanses your breath and makes your mouth feel refreshed. It also prevents the spread of viruses when used regularly.

♦ Luxury Foaming Bath

Bathing with mountains of pampering bubbles containing *T36-C7* and naturally moisturizing nut oils and herbs, this is a must for people with dry and sensitive skin.

♦ Mela-Gel

This form of Melaleuca is a pocket first aid kit in a jar. Because of its convenient container, I carry it wherever I go. The antiseptic qualities of *Melaleuca alternifolia* oil and the healing effects of vitamin E make this a perfect companion for anyone.

♦ Natural Shampoo

A refined and concentrated non-alkaline hair care product for regular usage, it can be utilized by the most sensitive skin.

♦ Natural Spa & Bath Oil

This absorptive formula made with oil of *Melaleuca alternifolia* soothes problem skin, relieves minor skin irritation and reduces the risk of infection. It is the natural oil squalene present in this product that makes it very healing to damaged or recovering skin.

♦ Nature's Cleanse

For candida yeast infections requiring a female douche, this product, when diluted, gives nearly instant relief. Very sensitive or irritated skin responds favorably to this buffered solution of oil of *Melaleuca alternifolia*. Follow the directions.

◆ Pain-A-Trate

For relieving muscle or joint aches and pains, there is no natural equal. *Pain-A-Trate* gives rapid relief to pain associated with osteoarthritis, bruises and injuries. *Pain-A-Trate* comes in two convenient forms: a cream and a lotion. *Caution! Pain-A-Trate* contains a natural form of aspirin. People who have experienced aspirin toxicity may react to this product.

◆ Problem Skin Lotion

For a protective moisturizer over wounds and injuries, this lotion is best applied after thoroughly cleansing the area.

◆ Sun-Shades All weather lotion

With a sun protective factor (SPF) 9, this highly protective barrier against hot and cold weather allows those who can tolerate some sun to get by without a total sun block. The ingredients of *T36-C7*, lanolins, herbal skin conditioners, delicate oils, and anti-oxidant vitamins makes this an excellent outdoor skin lotion.

◆ Sun-Shades Lip Balm

As a protective barrier against hot dry weather with an SPF of 15, this moisturizing product with oil of *Melaleuca alternifolia* provides maximum protection for the lips against the forces of nature.

◆ Sun-Shades Sport Waterproof Sunblock SPF 15

For people who are constantly outdoors, *Sun-Shades Sport Waterproof Sunblock SPF 15* prevents damage during prolonged exposure to the sun. Vegetable extracts, *T36-C7*, herbal skin conditioners, delicate oils, and anti-oxidant vitamins make this an excellent wet weather sunblock.

◆ Sun-Shades Max Waterproof Sunshield SPF 30

Maximum protection from cancer-causing ultraviolet radiation is achieved for infants and those with especially sensitive skin with *Sun-Shades Max Waterproof Sunshield SPF 30*. This product is formulated to provide the ultimate in wet weather protection.

◆ *T36-C7*

This product contains at least 36 per cent certified Terpenols and no more than 7 per cent Cineole. It has an antiseptic, analgesic, and cooling effect on skin. It is best used following the use of *Melaleuca Antibacterial Liquid Soap* to prevent infections. It also works very well in warm steam vaporizers. Caution - prolonged use to the same area can cause excessive drying.

◆ *T40-C5*

The most sensitive skin can use this product as an antiseptic, analgesic or skin stimulator. Green eyed redheads use this product with great results!

◆ *Triple Antibiotic Ointment*

This easy to use tube of concentrated ointment containing the oil of *Melaleuca alternifolia* and three highly effective antibiotics helps prevent and treat skin infections following injury. It gives lasting protection against most pathogenic bacteria, fungus, mold and viral infections.

◆ *Zap-It!*

For acne on the face, neck and back, this product blends the affects of *Melaleuca alternifolia* oil and the astringent benzoyl chloride. It is very effective for pimples.

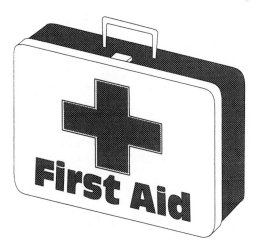

PERSONAL NOTES

◆ Access Bar

The process of storing fat and protecting it during famine or hibernation is caused by high levels of a metabolite called adenosine. When inhibitors of adenosine are supplied in the diet, as in the *Access Bar*, this helps the body release fat reserves for primary energy usage. One bar taken 15 minutes before physical exercise, helps burn fat in a natural and healthy way. This exceptional product is patented and satisfaction is guaranteed.

◆ Cell Wise Anti-Oxidants

One of the greatest breakthroughs in science has been the knowledge that plants manufacture substances to protect their chemistry against the suns harmful radiation and pollution. Amazingly, these same substances also protect animal cells against the same types of damage. Anti-oxidants, free radical scavengers, methyl donors and electron-rich poly cyclic compounds that prevent damage and premature aging of human cells are the major components in *Cell Wise Anti-Oxidants*.

◆ CounterAct

CounterAct Cold, Allergy Sinus Medicine contains three proven medicines for relief of cold or sinus congestion. Acetominophen is an aspirin-free analgesic, Phenylpropanolanine Hydrochloride is a powerful nasal decongestant, and Chlorpheniramine Maleate is a proven antihistamine. These ingredients combine for effective relief of the symptoms of sneezing, nasal congestion, and fever as well as pain relief. Occasional sinus, nasal, and upper chest congestion caused by seasonal hay fever or inhaled irritants is relieved effectively with *CounterAct Cold, Allergy Sinus Medicine.* *CounterAct Cough Relief Medicine* contains Guaifenesin a powerful expectorant to relieve chest congestion and Dextromethorphan Hydrobromide a cough suppressant. This formula contains no alcohol and will not make you drowsy.

♦ G'Day Melaleuca Herbal Tea

The *G'Day Melaleuca Tea*, made from the dried leaf, was the original form that Captain Cook discovered the native Australians using. Many nutritive factors are present in varying amounts including essential oils, water soluble vitamins, minerals, and antioxidants, as well as natural water soluble esters of terpene-3-ol's and terpene-4-ol's. These tend to have many beneficial effects on the digestive tract, circulation, elimination, nervous system and immune system.

♦ MEL-VITA

Three out of every four people fail to meet their daily needs of at least one known essential nutrient. *MEL-VITA*, with the addition of *Melaleuca alternifolia* leaf to help prevent colon accumulation of unfriendly microbes, is a unique multiple vitamin formula useful as added insurance against dietary deficiencies.

♦ MELA-CAL

Supplementation of extra calcium, magnesium, phosphorus, vitamins D and C for women, growing children and those who exercise is now advised by the surgeon general to build healthy bones, as well as prevent bone loss later in life. The addition of *Melaleuca alternifolia* leaf makes this formula unique.

♦ ProVex & ProVex-Plus

Why do plants never get cancer? This question has led to the discovery of phytochemicals of the flavonoid family of antho- and proanthocyanidins. Having 20-50 times the antioxidant effectiveness of vitamin E and Vitamin C, these special antioxidant formulas are designed for those individuals who may be taking *Cell Wise Anti-Oxidants,* but need additional protection against the damaging effects of free radicals. The added Ginkgo and Bilberry herbs give extra circulatory support to persons prone to cataracts or failing memory.

◆ Sustain Drink

Sudden energy loss during and after exercise or work, can be minimized by using this mixed carbohydrate beverage in place of sugary fruit juice or soda pop. It helps maintain energy and prevent electrolyte loss.

◆ This Is Fiber?

Lower calorie demands make it difficult to get enough soluble and insoluble fiber from our diet. This convenient low fat snack actually contributes valuable roughage to our diet which reduces absorption of certain pesticides, herbicides and dietary fats, and speeds bowel transit of food wastes which aids regularity.

◆ Vita-Bears

Children's chewable vitamins and minerals should be formulated to meet the unique challenges of growth, physical and mental development. This formula meets those needs with the addition of fructose compounding to insure maximum absorption and *Melaleuca alternifolia* leaf to control unfriendly microbe growth in the digestive tract. Getting young children trained to supplement their diet early in life is easy. Don't wait until they are teenagers!

◆ Vitality Pak

MEL-VITA, *MELA-CAL*, and *Cell Wise Anti-Oxidants* when taken together are a basic daily nutritional ration. These three products complement each other and work together to boost the healing capacity of the body.

PERSONAL NOTES

◆ *ClearPower*

ClearPower leaves your windows and mirrors with a shine and streak-free. *ClearPower* is very concentrated and economical. It is environmentally safe and biodegradable.

◆ *Diamond Brite*

If I were on a deserted island with a sink full of dishes and a dishwasher, my one wish would be to have a bottle of *Diamond Brite*. This is the best there is. You will find that there will not be a yucky film on your dishes that you taste with each bite of food.

◆ *MelaDrops*

Your dishes will come out of the sink with a beautiful shine to them after washing in *MelaDrops*. *MelaDrops* is very concentrated so only a few drops will do the job.

◆ *MelaMagic*

MelaMagic works very well on the toughest of jobs. It cleans everything from ovens to sidewalks. *MelaMagic* is highly concentrated and economical.

◆ *MelaPower*

This is the best antiseptic laundry detergent anywhere. *MelaPower* is pH balanced and non-alkaline to preserve fabric strength and color. *MelaPower* is highly concentrated and biodegradable.

◆ *MelaSoft*

Say good bye to static and hello to soft clothes. *MelaSoft* is very concentrated so use only a few sprays in the dryer or a capful in the washer.

◆ *Pre-Spot*

My neighbor cannot believe how clean and spotless looking my families clothes come out of the wash. *Pre-Spot* is bleach and phosphate free. It does not contain harsh acids and is non-aerosol. It gets even the worst stains out completely.

♦ Sol-U-Mel

This water-soluble emulsion of oil of *Melaleuca alternifolia* is used to enhance the disinfectant and cleaning properties of other products. When diluted, it can be used on the skin or in general cleaning or laundry duties. *Sol-U-Mel* removes road tar, chewing gum, motor oil, and other stains from any surface. It will deodorize and sanitize rooms and counters, as well as clothing and fabrics. *Sol-U-Mel* is environmentally safe.

♦ Tough 'N Tender

Tough 'N Tender is made to be tough on dirt and grease, yet gentle on your hands. It is highly concentrated and very versatile in its use.

♦ Tub 'N Tile

You will see rust disappear before your eyes when using *Tub 'N Tile*. It is made from organic acids, derived from sugar cane. You can clean brass and copper as well as your bathroom sink, tub, and anything else that looks a bit rusty.

♦   These products are trademarks of Melaleuca, Inc, Idaho Falls, ID.

VITALITY FOR LIFE
PERSONAL HEALTH RISK APPRAISAL

Health knowledge is gained through education and personal experience. The literal meaning of the word doctor is *"teacher"* or helper in the constant struggle to maintain wellness and prevent disease. Some societies pay doctors to keep citizens healthy and make the doctors treat patients for free when they become sick. This prevents any doctor from ever being accused of trying to keep his patient sick for personal economic reasons or from experimenting at the patient's expense. Unfortunately, many of our doctors see themselves as technicians (specialists) and merely *"repair"* or *"replace"* body parts once they fail to function. *"That's not my specialty - let me refer you to someone else."* Others often use dangerous drugs to control the symptoms with no hope given of overcoming the illness . The cost in the number of unproductive citizens, as well as dollars, because of *"treating"* conditions is staggering. This standard of *"disease care"* offers no end in sight. The individual citizen must become active in the pursuit for health rather than being passive and waiting until a disease develops. Such is the purpose behind a program like the *Vitality For Life Personal Health Risk Appraisal* - to make you aware of your weaknesses and direct your attention toward means to prevent the inevitable from happening. Society will soon be unable to pay the tab.

I was very pleased to see the Melaleuca company introduce the *Vitality For Life Personal Health Risk Appraisal* in 1993. We have been performing a similar analysis with blood chemistry analysis, physical examination, lifestyle and diet analysis for over 15 years. Our patients have proven how effective natural alternatives can be. Like the motor oil commercial says, *"You can pay me now (for an oil change), or you can pay me later (for an overhaul.)"* Many of you who have visited our clinic have expressed the need for more of this type of education in other parts of the country. Now it is available to many more North Americans thanks to the Melaleuca company. You may want to track your regular *Vitality For Life Personal Health Risk Appraisals* in the appendix provided at the end of this book. This gives you a quick reference and visual means of seeing just how far you have come.

For people who want to know how to implement prevention into their daily life, we have over 100 educational video and audio tape titles available. These tapes cover most common health concerns, ranging from Acne to Yeast Infections. We encourage you to use this educational resource to learn more about your particular health concern. Appendix 4 in this book has a listing of some of the available titles. For a free catalog of available video and audio tapes call (800) 845-2025.

Vitality For Life Personal Health Risk Appraisal Log

The following chart is for you to record the scores from your *Vitality For Life Personal Health Risk Appraisal*s.

Test Dates				
Overall Health Risk				
Coronary Risk Profile				
Cancer Risk Profile				
Body Composition Profile				
Nutrition Profile				
Stress Profile				
Safety Profile				
Lifestyle Profile				
Exercise Profile				
Health Risk Age				
Chronological Age				
Achievable Risk Age				

COMMON HEALTH CONDITIONS

The following section provides self-help guidelines for common health conditions. These recommendations are based on medical research and my 20 years experience with *Melaleuca Alternifolia* oil. If you have specific questions not addressed in this book, first consult *HEALTH TALK*, my free 24 hour health advisor. If you still have questions, please call the clinic to schedule a time for a telephone consultation. See Appendix for further details.

It is recommended that you develop a good relationship with a physician knowledgeable in the art and science of natural and preventive medicine. The information in this book is not a substitute for the care you should be receiving from your primary physician. In all cases involving a physical or medical complaint, please consult your physician.

ABDOMINAL DISTRESS

The area between the pelvis and the rib cage contains more organs and more sites for discomfort than any other area of the body. Colic or upset stomach in infants, indigestion, reactions to foods, and constipation are common problems which can occur. The bowel, liver, pancreas, kidneys, spleen, stomach, and gall bladder are all possible sites of distress.

Of all abdominal distress, gas and indigestion account for 80% of complaints. Abdominal distress is often caused by unhealthy eating habits. While we should all drink at least eight glasses of pure water a day, this water should be consumed between meals rather than at meal time. When we drink too many liquids with our meal, digestive enzymes are diluted. This, in turn, can be manifested as indigestion or abdominal pain caused by bloating and gas.

Upon feeling discomfort in the abdomen, one should try to remember if food was ingested which was of questionable freshness. The so-called *summer flu* which many experience is actually due to bacterial toxicity from improperly handled food.

Overeating in the evening hours or eating in a hurry packs food in the stomach before nerve and hormone stimulation can properly begin the digestive process. Eating rich, fatty meals stresses the stomach, gallbladder and pancreas which slows down digestion and allows ever-present bacteria to begin fermentation and putrefaction in the bowel.

Constipation is at epidemic levels in our country. Eating high roughage foods helps hold moisture in the bowel, giving the muscles of the bowel physical material to propel along its some 26 feet. This roughage rapidly carries ingested toxins, proliferating bacteria, and metabolic byproducts out of the body. Experts agree that 20 to 30 grams of roughage per day is advisable for adults. As a result of a mechanized and refined food lifestyle, the average American eats 7.3 grams of roughage each day. For more information, call *HEALTH TALK* and consult topics 41 through 47.

TREATMENT: Celebrate eating. Give thanks. Eat as many meals with soft music and candle light in the presence of people you love as possible. Drink adequate amounts of liquid including 2 or 3 cups of *G'Day Melaleuca Tea* each day - between meals. Slow down! Use *This Is Fiber?* bars to supplement your daily intake of roughage. Get 20 to 40 minutes of moderate daily exercise to promote circulation within the abdomen and stimulate bowel peristalsis. Multiple small meals are generally preferable to one or two large meals each day. To correct colic in infants, give several teaspoons of warm *G'Day Melaleuca Tea* during the day and before bed. Take *The Vitality Pak* daily to encourage proper metabolism and waste excretion from cells.

ABRASIONS

These injuries occur when your skin slides across course materials, such as concrete, gravel or asphalt. The top layers of skin are damaged causing nerves, blood vessels and lymph vessels to be exposed to the air. This causes immediate pain and creates an opportunity for germs to enter the body. After the bleeding and oozing stops, a dry protective scab will usually form within a few hours and is nature's protection against infection.

TREATMENT: Washing the area gently yet thoroughly with the *Antibacterial Liquid Soap* and cool water quickly reduces the pain. (Warm or hot water increases nerve stimulation and pain in most people.) Allow the stream of water to wash off all visible particulates. Pick out any embedded material. (If pure water is not available, douse the area thoroughly with *T36-C7* to sanitize. Cover with *Antibacterial Liquid Soap* or *Problem Skin Lotion* keeping the wound soft until water and cleansing of debris is possible.) Apply *Triple Antibiotic Ointment* or *Mela-Gel* and allow to remain open to the air if possible. Otherwise, use a loose bandage saturated with *Triple Antibiotic Ointment* or *Mela-Gel* to prevent sticking. Repeat administration of *Triple Antibiotic Ointment* or *Mela-Gel* as frequently as needed for several days until the wound is adequately covered with a scab.

ABSCESSES

These painful, pus filled sacks of infection can occur in or on any surface of the body. I have treated abscesses on the head, neck, chest, leg, armpit, nose, anus, vagina, and inside of the mouth. Abscesses may start from a cut, scratch, pimple, ingrown hair, ingrown finger nail or toenail, hemorrhoid or pierced ears for ear rings. Occasionally the lack of proper treatment of an infection can produce the characteristic swollen, red, painful lump. The typical bacteria which causes abscesses is *Staph. epidermis* which is found on healthy skin. While antibiotics are often necessary, the overuse of antibiotics either by prescription, or in the meat we eat, has led to the development of many antibiotic resistant strains of bacteria. For more information, call *HEALTH TALK* and consult topics 18 and 22.

TREATMENT: Begin drinking *G'Day Melaleuca Tea* in place of other liquids 3 to 4 times each day. Apply *T36-C7* to the abscess. To encourage drainage and drive the *T36-C7* into the wound, apply hot moist packs over the area. If the abscess can be lanced and drained, soak afterward in solution of 1 oz *Sol-U-Mel* and 2 Tbs. of Epsom salts in 1 quart of warm water. If the area is unable to be soaked, saturate a hand towel in the solution, wring it out, heat in a microwave for 1 minute then apply to the affected area for 10 minutes. Repeat every hour to speed draining. Apply *Triple Antibiotic Ointment* or *Mela-Gel*. If needed, cover with gauze to absorb any seeping fluid and keep the area clean.

ACNE

Overproduction of the oil glands in the skin can dry and harden, forming blackheads. These may produce a local bacterial infection and pimples. Acne is common to those working in hostile chemical environments, people suffering with hormonal imbalances or those under physical or emotional stress. Skin blemishes in these individuals arise from improper nutrition, toxicity, and rapidly changing needs for hormonal regulation. Familial or lifestyle traits are learned from our parents and often give the appearance of a genetic link. Our patients from 10 to 70 years of age with this problem have gotten wonderful results using a combination of factors. For more information, call *HEALTH TALK* and consult topics 16 and 17. You may wish to see my educational video tape titled Acne.

TREATMENT: Suspect food allergies and experiment with elimination diets or get tested by a natural physician. Minimize sugar. Drink 3 to 4 cups of *G'Day Melaleuca Tea,* hot or iced each day, in addition to the regular 8 glasses of pure water you should normally drink. Reduce fats to less than 20% of total calories. Perspire for 20 minutes each day, preferably from exercise, but sauna or steam baths work also. Shower while washing entire body with *Antibacterial Liquid Soap* or *Gold Bar* and a soft wash cloth. For those who prefer bathing, always put 1 oz of *Sol-U-Mel* in the tub. Especially avoid eating cooked oils such as margarine and potato chips. Get 20 grams of fiber including a *This Is Fiber?* bar daily. Take *MEL-VITA* with every meal for the added nutrient benefits of vitamin A, zinc, B vitamins and vitamin C. Apply *Zap-It!* or *T36-C7* to any developing pustule. Apply *T36-C7* to blackheads to

clear the plugged oil duct. Apply *Problem Skin Lotion* **afterward to keep moisture in skin and resist oil accumulation. Avoid dry brush or friction rubs with alcohol as this naturally stimulates oil production. Get enough rest.**

AIR PURIFICATION

The quality of the air you breathe in your home may be robbing you of good health. Modern energy efficient homes, by virtue of their air-tight design, often trap chemical vapors from furniture, carpets and building cements, in addition to mold, fungus, yeast and bacteria from moist condensation in heating and cooling air ducts, soil from house plants and under sink areas. There is a literal zoo co-inhabiting in our homes. Many respiratory, eye, ear, nose and throat complaints appear in my waiting room because of over-exposure to foul household air. Changes of seasons often shift populations of these microbial species as growing conditions fluctuate. One man said, *"I can count on a sore throat and itching eyes the first week we start the furnace in the Fall."* For more information, call *HEALTH TALK* and consult topics 33 through 38.

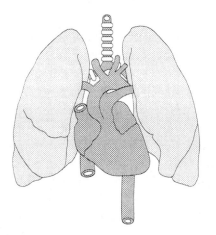

TREATMENT: Use only biologically safe cleaners in your home. Remove browning leaves from house plants immediately. Do not over-water house plants and provide good drainage. Change furnace and cooling air return filters

monthly during extreme weather usage. To do a Melaleuca oil purge of your house two to twelve times a year, attach an inverted open bottle of *T36-C7* on the furnace intake filter. The high air volume will diffuse the entire contents of the bottle throughout your house over the next 12 to 36 hours (depending upon temperature and relative humidity). This treated air flows throughout all the rooms and stops the growth of bacteria, molds, fungus and viruses. Take *ProVex* or *ProVex-Plus* when exposed to toxic substances.

ALLERGIC REACTIONS

Skin rashes, itching skin, sore throat, runny nose, sinus congestion, eye irritation, headaches, and fatigue are common symptoms of allergy sufferers. While individuals vary in their degree of sensitivity to allergic substances, it is important to minimize discomfort and prevent complications such as infections. Many of the aromatic oils from *Melaleuca alternifolia* have local acting anti-inflammatory and desensitization effects. A number of my patients have experienced relief from contact allergens, air borne allergens and even food allergens while following some simple advice. You may wish to see my educational video tape on Allergies.

TREATMENT: Always try to avoid the allergen when possible. Your natural physician can help you determine the substances you are reacting to and begin a program to gain permanent desensitization. Applying *T36-C7* directly to exposed skin reaction sites (hands, arms, legs, feet, scalp, neck and abdomen area) usually neutralizes the local histamine reaction and reduces symptoms. A word of caution - do not apply any *Melaleuca* products near or in the eyes. Avoid rubbing the affected skin to prevent further irritation. *Problem Skin Lotion* or *Mela-Gel* can be applied afterwards to give long lasting protection. Soaking in a bath containing 1 oz of *Natural Spa & Bath Oil* (and 1 oz of *Sol-U-Mel* if infections are present) offers an added soothing effect. Remember, allergies are the result of an unhealthy immune system, so maximizing your nutrition is essential. Besides eating wholesome foods, *MEL-VITA* and

Cell Wise Anti-Oxidants taken with every meal gives extra protection against allergies by providing anti-oxidants in the form of beta carotene, vitamin C, and vitamin E (Anti-oxidants reduce histamine levels which cause the itching, rashing and burning). The calcium in *MELA-CAL* often gives immediate relief from sneezing and general body aches during a reaction. When your nose and throat are affected by hay fever, dust, pollen, or food reactions, breathing hot steam from either a vaporizer or bowl of steaming water with 5 drops of *T36-C7* each morning and evening for 15 to 20 minutes gives a welcome relief.

ANEMIA

Insufficient red blood cells and/or hemoglobin causes fatigue and lack of motivation. *Blood loss* due to hemorrhage somewhere within the body or *decreased production* of red blood cells are the two sources. There are several varied conditions which result in anemia. Iron deficiency due to poor nutrition is most common in teenage girls and the elderly. Heavy menstrual flow is often associated with anemia. Drugs such as aspirin thin the blood and cause micro-hemorrhage in the gastrointestinal tract. This can cause anemia, especially in women who use this medication for menstrual pain and cramps. Copper, zinc, protein, and B vitamins are essential for a healthy supply of red blood cells. Deficiencies of any of these can lead to various types of anemia which are often difficult to diagnose. A sudden drop in red blood cells (hemolytic anemia) or hemoglobin (hypochromic anemia) is one of the early warning signs of cancer. Infestation of bowel parasites from outdoor pets can also lead to anemia and malnutrition. Often, anemias can only be clearly identified by a complete blood chemistry and blood cell study. Your natural physician can provide further information regarding anemias. You may wish to see my educational video tape titled Anemia.

TREATMENT: Avoid over-the-counter drugs. Ask your doctor about the side effects of any prescription medications. Eat an adequate amount of green vegetables, whole grains, fish, poultry and a small amount of red meat. Take *The Vitality Pak* regularly to supplement iron and essential nutrients to insure adequate red blood cell building blocks.

Drink 2 cups of *G'Day Melaleuca Tea* each day to maximize kidney detoxification. Get 20 minutes of moderate exercise five times each week to adequately oxygenate the body.

ANTISEPTICS

An ounce of prevention is worth a pound of cure when it comes to germs that cause infection. Any break in the skin is a potential site for infection. Use protective gear, clothing, boots, hats, back braces or goggles when needed.

PREVENTIVE TREATMENT: Bathe or shower with *Antibacterial Liquid Soap* or *Gold Bar* which leaves a fine layer of Melaleuca oil on the skin. For jobs where your hands will become dirty, use *Sol-U-Mel* or *Antibacterial Liquid Soap* as a preventive hand glove. If an injury occurs, there is a barrier of between you and the awaiting germs. You can simply rinse the pre-treated area with warm water and lift the germs off with the soap. Apply *Problem Skin Lotion* afterward. This is especially good for mechanics to prevent grease and grime (often loaded with germs) from forcing its way into the skin. It is also especially effective around farm machinery and animals.

APPENDICITIS

Pain in the lower right abdomen which causes a bent posture and an elevated white blood cell count are sufficient evidence to wheel a person into surgery and remove the appendix - just before it bursts! The human appendix is a lymphatic collector of wastes protecting the valve between the small and large intestine. Its purpose is not clearly known, but it carries a reputation of getting infected and being the cause of many failed human endeavors. When studying human anatomy in dissection class, I was amazed to see that some people had scars on their vermiform appendices. I asked the professor what was the cause of this. He said that many people have minor infections and even ruptures of their appendix (stomach aches, colic or *"flu"* symptoms) but totally recover to finish their lifetime.

Some, obviously, do not survive. Apparently, food and bacteria can lodge in the appendix and breed putrefaction and infection. Constipation commonly precedes appendicitis. For more information, call *HEALTH TALK* and consult topics 39-47 and 94. See the section on Abdominal Distress in this book.

TREATMENT: Prevention is the best solution. Drink 2 to 4 quarts of liquids including water, *G'Day Melaleuca Tea*, and juices each day. I frequently recommend, and practice, drinking hot water upon rising each morning to get the system primed and hydrated. Exercise moderately at least 5 days each week. Get 30 grams of soluble and insoluble roughage each day including *This Is Fiber?* to prevent constipation. Remember - healthy people typically have a bowel movement within 2 hours after EACH meal!

ARMS/LEGS ASLEEP

Loss of feeling in the arms or legs (paraesthesia) can be caused from a temporary pinch of a nerve while sleeping or having someone sit on your lap. It also can be progressive due to peripheral circulatory problems where the sensory nerves in the extremities do not receive enough blood. We have seen people who have handled toxic solvents, paints, cleaners, pesticides or herbicides and soon after experience extremity paraesthesia. One man bought a retail business one winter and decided to save money painting and wallpapering it himself. After breathing and handling the paint and cleaners for two weeks in the heated but improperly ventilated space, he started waking with numbness in his feet and fingers which did not disappear. Six weeks after the painting was finished, he came to my office in great despair. He couldn't feel a sheet of paper when held between his fingers or use stairs without a light. A true case of neurotoxicity. For more information, call *HEALTH TALK* and consult topics 11, 49 and 54-62. You may wish to see my educational video tape on Detoxification.

TREATMENT: If you are susceptible to paraesthesias, do not try to sleep in a moving vehicle without an inflatable cushion behind your neck. Trade legs often when holding someone on your lap. Be checked by a chiropractor when you have

any kind of traumatic accident to your neck or back. Use *Pain-A-Trate* on any tender muscles in your neck and upper back. Always have adequate ventilation when using volatile solvents or paint. Remember - at first your nose will alert you to the danger. If unheeded, the signal will diminish until you *"get used to it"*. Use only environmentally safe sprays. *ProVex* or *ProVex-Plus* should be taken daily. Take *The Vitality Pak* every few hours to offset the destruction of nutrients by these substances in your liver. Take *This Is Fiber?* to carry the substances out of your digestive tract quickly. Drink extra water, *G'Day Melaleuca Tea* and the *Sustain Drink* for maintaining blood sugar during environmentally stressful times. Exercise after an exposure to harsh volatile chemicals to flush the lungs. Sweat from exercise or in a sauna or steam bath to wash out as many toxins as possible.

ARTHRITIS

Hot, red, painful and stiff swollen joints of the hands, wrists, elbows, neck, back, hips, and knees are common symptoms of arthritis. The mummified Pharaohs suffered with this malady. More remedies are sold to treat arthritis than any other common condition. Arthritis can be caused by old injuries, allergies, gout, mineral deficiencies, hyperactive immune response, toxicity, poor circulation, handling of cold goods or prescription drug side effects. Further information is found in my educational video tape on Arthritis.

TREATMENT: The best long term treatment is the one that gets at the cause. Some cases of arthritis respond to reducing white sugar, white flour, nicotine, caffeine, and alcohol. Generally avoid cold temperatures to the affected joint. Some forms of arthritis respond well to resting the joint while other forms, such as osteoarthritis, respond to motion such as knitting. *Pain-A-Trate* and *T36-C7* can be applied to the affected area with a heating pad or hot moist pack to achieve rapid relief of pain and stiffness. Some elderly patients do this every morning as faithfully as eating their prunes. *ProVex* or *ProVex-Plus* should be taken daily. Taking *The Vitality Pak* with each meal provides essential trace nutrients for reducing further injury and increasing healing. Dehydrated joints ache, therefore, drink more liquids including 2 to 4 cups of *G'Day Melaleuca Tea* per day.

ASTHMA

Congestion and restriction of the lungs causes labored breathing and wheezing and affects one out of every twelve people. Many are small children. Although it is associated with airborne allergies and occasional food sensitivities, improvement can occur by following a few simple suggestions. See the section on Chest Congestion in this book. For more information, call *HEALTH TALK* and consult topic 38.

TREATMENT: Identify and restrict all sensitizing substances (See Air Purification). Adults can try adding 10 to 20 drops of Tabasco sauce (capsicum) in a few ounces of water and drinking it immediately before a meal to reduce congestion and thin mucous in the lungs. One drop of *T36-C7* on a cotton tipped swab gently used to clean pollen and dust from each nostril before bed has helped many children in our practice. Take *The Vitality Pak* with each meal for adults and *Vita-Bears* with each meal for children to increase resistance to attacks. Apply *Pain-A-Trate* to the chest of adults and children before bed. Get enough rest. If congestion exists, use *CounterAct,* 1 tablet 3-4 times per day.

ATHEROSCLEROSIS

Hardening of the arteries can lead to high blood pressure, shortness of breath, strokes, cold hands and feet, as well as senility and premature aging. Cholesterol (LDL - the bad kind) and ionic calcium make up part of the *"cement"* which lines arteries of the liver, bowel, lungs, brain, kidneys, legs and arms. Several common sense suggestions can help.

TREATMENT: Stop smoking and avoid smokers. Have a *Vitality For Life Personal Health Risk Appraisal* performed to determine your risks. Chart your progress in the Appendix of this book. Avoid animal fats and cooked vegetable fats. Reduce total fat to less than 20% of your total diet. Eat 2 servings of raw or stewed fruit along with 5 servings of green, yellow and orange colored vegetables each day. Begin a gradual daily exercise program. Eat an *Access Bar* 15 minutes before exercising and drink *Sustain Drink* one half hour after exercising to speed up the fat burning process. Take *The Vitality Pak* with every meal. Take *ProVex* or *ProVex-Plus* daily. Drink 3 to 4 cups of *G'Day Melaleuca Tea* daily.

ATHLETE'S FOOT

Public showers offer a great opportunity to contact the fungus which causes *tinea pedis*, known as athlete's foot. Blistering often occurs when the immune system becomes sensitized to the fungus. When the fungus infects the upper body, this is known as *tinea corporis*, or ringworm, causing raised and reddened rashes with clear centers. Long term athlete's foot often involves the toenails and often totally destroys the nail plate and may enter the bone. This infection will persist indefinitely until treatment is effective. The general health of the individual tends to determine the magnitude of the infection and extent of the symptoms. For more information, call *HEALTH TALK* and consult topics 20, 62, 88 and 95.

TREATMENT: As in most infections, prevention is the best treatment. Always wear shower sandals when in public showers such as athletic locker rooms and swimming pools Also, apply *T36-C7*, *Mela-Gel* or *Triple Antibiotic Ointment* between toes and to bottoms of feet immediately after showering. Direct sunlight and air drying the feet after showering or swimming is also a helpful preventive measure. Take *The Vitality Pak* with each meal to optimize trace nutrients. Drink 2 to 3 cups of *G'Day Melaleuca Tea* daily. The following suggestions have produced favorable results in eliminating athlete's foot. Bathing is advised over showering. Use 1 oz of *Sol-U-Mel* along with *Natural Spa & Bath Oil* in the tub. Use a clean washcloth with the *Antibacterial Liquid Soap* or *Gold Bar*. Drink 2 to 6 cups of *G'Day Melaleuca Tea* daily. Apply *T36-C7* to any active or itching areas. Allow it to dry before applying *Mela-Gel* or *Triple Antibiotic Ointment*. Cracking or oozing skin should receive a generous amount of *Problem Skin Lotion*. Take *The Vitality Pak* of nutritional supplements regularly.

ATHLETIC INJURIES

The human body is designed for motion. Actually, everyone is an athlete - You are either actively practicing or you are not. More middle aged and elderly people are enjoying the benefits of regular exercise than ever before. Typical athletic injuries in all ages include pulled muscles, strained ligaments and tendons, bruises and muscle cramps. I can say that as I near a half century of life, I have more aches and pains if I don't exercise daily than if I do. I will always strive to be an amateur racket ball player, weight lifter and runner - even with my injuries. Of course, proper warm up and cool down, and stretching before and after working out is essential, but what can we do to prevent so many *owies*? For more information on preventing and caring for athletic injuries, call *HEALTH TALK* and consult topics 6, 10, 58-62 and 97. See the sections on Abrasions, Bruises and Cuts in this book.

TREATMENT: Take *The Vitality Pak* every meal to optimize tissue strengthening trace nutrients. Take more *MELA-CAL* if you have muscle cramps after a work out. Eat an *Access Bar* 15 minutes before exercise to inhibit adenosine and open fat stores in the body for energy. *Sustain Drink* can be mixed in your water bottle for continual replenishment of waning blood sugar. *Pain-A-Trate* should be in the equipment bag of every athlete. Regular application of *T36-C7* stimulates circulation to injured tissue. Immediate application of *Pain-A-Trate* to any closed injury will start the healing process. Ice is good for injured joints, muscles, tendons and ligaments. Apply ice for no more than 5 to 10 minutes at a time. Longer treatment periods can actually cause frostbite or reverse the anti-inflammatory effect. Heat can cause problems so it should be avoided, in most cases, for the first 24 to 48 hours after an injury to bruised or pulled muscles. Chronic or untreated injuries that do not resolve should be seen by a chiropractor or physician trained to treat sports injuries. Take *ProVex* or *ProVex-Plus* daily to heal damaged tissues.

BABY TEETH

All 20 baby teeth are usually present by the age of 4. Children will loose these teeth from the ages of 5 to 12 as the size of the growing head and mouth require larger teeth. Care and protection of these teeth is important to insure a healthy environment for the permanent teeth which must last 75 years.

TREATMENT: Do not put a child to bed with a nursing bottle of fruit juice. This is the most common cause of *"dissolved"* baby teeth and the need for capping. Teach the 2 year old to brush with *Dental Gel for Kids*, with supervision, after every meal. The younger they learn, the longer it lasts. Give your child *Vita-Bears* to insure strong healthy teeth.

BACK PAIN

More than one half of the adult American population suffers with back pain. Our sedentary lifestyle, motorized transportation, and poor diets cause a large portion of our discomfort. Being a chiropractor, I see many people who are suffering needlessly. Stretching and strengthening exercises, eating a healthy diet, maintaining our healthy weight, supplementing calcium, magnesium, and micro-nutrients, and correcting spinal injuries before they become chronic can go a long way towards reducing back pain. For more information, call *HEALTH TALK* and consult topic 55. You may wish to see my educational video tape on Back Pain.

TREATMENT: Apply *Pain-A-Trate* to over-worked muscles. Apply moderate heat (use cold immediately after injury or acute pain 5 to 10 minutes each hour for first 6 to 24 hours before using heat). Use *T36-C7* on skin over spasming back muscles to promote the relaxation reflex. Take *MELA-CAL* every 2 to 4 hours to relax muscles. Drink 2 to 4 cups of *G'Day Melaleuca Tea* each day. Take *ProVex* or *ProVex-Plus* daily to help heal collagen structures in your back.

BARBER'S ITCH

Caused by a fungus from an improperly cleaned razor, shaving cream brush or electric shaver, the typical reddened rash is less common since the use of disposable razors and canned shaving foam or gel. See the sections on Athlete's Foot in this book.

BATHING

One of the most self pampering events of life is taking a hot bath. Getting the most out of your time and effort is essential. Depending upon your desire for temperature, bubbles and relaxation time, bathing is ideal for body self examination as well as meditation and mental cool down. Showers expose persons with respiratory or skin sensitivities to 8 to 10 times the amount of chlorine as bathing. Chlorine sensitive persons should run hot bath water and allow it to degas for about 5 minutes with the window open or the vent fan running before plunging in. Never take long baths (30 minutes or more) with a breeze in the room, as the lungs are susceptible to infections from cool air when the body is heated above 100 degrees. Put *Sol-U-Mel* (1 oz per tub) in the water to thoroughly sanitize and disinfect the skin. The *Natural Spa & Bath Oil* or the *Luxury Foaming Bath* are real therapy for the pores of the skin. See the sections on Sauna Baths and Hot Tubs in this book.

BED SORES

Also known as decubitus ulcers, bed sores occur when people are bedfast or confined to a wheel chair. A lambs wool or *"egg carton"* foam pad can be placed under the person to prevent the deep crater sores from forming. Daily inspection is important to identify the blanched skin heralding the onset of a bedsore. Once started, bed sores can lead to infections and delayed healing. Prevention is the best treatment.

TREATMENT: Healing begins at the outer edges and works inward. Apply *T36-C7* to any blanched skin areas before the sore begins. It can often be halted at this stage. If a sore is present, gently wash the area with a washcloth and *Antibacterial Liquid Soap* enriched with a quarter ounce (1 capful) of *Sol-U-Mel* in 1 quart of warm water. Apply *Triple Antibiotic Ointment.* Cover with a loose gauze. Use minimum amount of tape. Repeat washing and *Triple Antibiotic Ointment* every 8 hours until the wound heals, which can be from one day to several weeks depending upon the overall health of the individual. NOTE: Bed sores should be taken very seriously in diabetics, persons on immune suppressive drugs, and those with leg ulcers due to poor circulation.

BEE AND WASP STINGS

Bees are territorial creatures. They defend their territory by injecting a powerful chemical, formic acid, into the intruder. This injection also contains traces of immune reactive agents that can provoke violent reactions in humans.

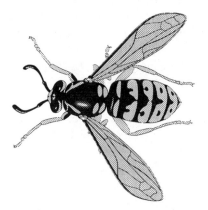

TREATMENT: Carefully remove the stinger by scraping it out. Wash the area with *Antibacterial Liquid Soap* and cold water. Immediately apply *T36-C7* or *Mela-Gel* to stop pain and prevent secondary infection. Do not use any other home remedies, such as baking soda with the Melaleuca products in this treatment. Reapply every 15 minutes until all signs and symptoms are gone. Four to six treatments may be necessary. Take *ProVex* or *ProVex-Plus* immediately and continue for 24 hours. NOTE: When a person is allergic to bee or wasp stings, this can be life threatening. The allergic person should carry an antidote kit containing adrenaline and benedryl. Administer this according to the directions before any other therapy. Shortness of breath or difficulty breathing, puffy or swollen throat or eyes, rapid heart rate, dizziness, or profuse sweating are signs of allergic reaction and can appear within 10 to 30 minutes after being stung. *DO NOT DELAY, GET EMERGENCY HELP!*

BLACK EYE

Bruising almost anywhere on the head resulting from an auto accident, reaching for the last cookie (just kidding) or even extensive dental work can cause a black eye.

TREATMENT: Apply an ice pack as soon as possible after the injury, to slow down facial swelling. Do <u>not</u> use *Mela-Gel* or *T36-C7* near the eye, as its aromatic vapor is drying to the eye and causes pain.

BLADDER INFECTIONS

Bladder infections, most often in women, can be bothersome at least and a potential full-blown illness at worst. Panties made of synthetic fabric cause excessive perspiration in women, which leads to bacterial growth at the opening of the urethra. Not drinking enough water encourages bacteria to grow within the urethra and bladder. Repeated infections is a cause for alarm. Note: Recurrent infections treated with antibiotics can lead to highly resistant strains of bacteria.

TREATMENT: Drink 2 to 6 cups of *G'Day Melaleuca Tea* along with 2-4 quarts of pure water each day. Wear cotton panties. Douche with *Nature's Cleanse* weekly to reduce bacteria in the area. Put 1 oz of *Sol-U-Mel* in rinse water of washing cycle when laundering undergarments.

BLEEDING

Bleeding from an open wound should receive immediate attention. Pulsating bleeding or spraying blood from a wound is an indication of a cut artery. Get trained emergency help immediately.

TREATMENT: Apply direct finger or hand pressure to the area sufficient to stop the bleeding. Elevate the body part above the heart if the bleeding is on an arm or leg. When the bleeding has stopped, apply *T36-C7, Triple Antibiotic Ointment,* or *Mela-Gel* under a pressure bandage to prevent infection and prevent the bandage from sticking to the wound. Change dressing every day until healing forms a dense scab. Do not apply *Pain-A-Trate*, as it contains natural aspirin which can prevent blood from clotting naturally.

BLEEDING GUMS

Deep plaque or periodontal infections can cause bleeding gums, swollen gums or dental pain. Brushing too hard is a common cause. Chronic vitamin C deficiency, alveolar (jaw) bone loss or chemical poisoning are other possible causes. The mouth is the literal window to overall health of the body!

TREATMENT: Regular brushing with *Tooth Polish* and rinsing with *Breath-Away* Mouthwash is a good way to control the build up of bacteria causing plaque. Daily flossing with *Dental Tape with T36-C7* can clean between teeth where a brush cannot reach. Drinking 2 to 4 cups of *G'Day Melaleuca Tea* per day helps promote a healthy environment in the mouth. Take *The Vitality Pak* and eat healthily. Get professional dental care if bleeding, pain or swelling of gums persists.

BLISTERS

Friction, chemical, or heat injuries can cause blistering which may lead to blood poisoning if not properly treated. For more information, call *HEALTH TALK* and consult topic 22.

TREATMENT: Do not puncture blisters. They can easily become infected. Mother Nature's band aid is the best. Immediately apply *T36-C7* to a developing blister. Ice is often helpful also. This will usually prevent further development. If the blister has formed, apply *Pain-A-Trate*, *Mela-Gel* or *Triple Antibiotic Ointment* and a cushioned bandage. The fluid pressure should reduce within 6 to 12 hours. Repeat treatment daily until the overlying skin sags, breaks open on its own and is replaced by a non-sensitive layer of skin from below. As long as there is pain, swelling or redness, continue treatment.

BODY LICE

Seeing a louse on a piece of clothing is one thing, seeing it on yourself or a friend is something else. Many parents, teachers and school nurses have contacted me because of my earlier book describing the Melaleuca oil treatment for Head Lice. Melaleuca oil products are a safe alternative to the prescription drug, lindane, as testified by many of you.

Lice infestation (Pediculosis) involves the head (P. capitus), the trunk or extremities (P. corporis), or the genital area (P. pubis). Originally, body lice prefer birds and almost any hairy mammal other than man. They will settle for second best (humans) when a warm puppy or chicken is absent but will selectively crawl to these animals if given a choice. (Humans smell bad to many parasites - Oh well, *"Any Port In A Storm."*) The louse lives directly off of blood after biting and puncturing the skin hence it can easily spread a multitude of diseases. It lives in hairy areas including eyebrows, eyelashes or beards where it lays its grayish-white eggs (nits) which can be seen with a magnifying glass on the hair follicles. The eggs hatch in three to fourteen days where the sluggish overweight looking insects seem eager for their first meal. Multiple families of lice cause excruciating pain, irritation and itching. They are

37

transmitted by contact with objects such as combs, hats, and shared garments. For this reason it is common among school children.

TREATMENT: Immediately upon suspecting or seeing evidence of lice, shampoo with *Natural Shampoo* and bathe in a mixture of 1 oz of *Sol-U-Mel* and 1 oz of *Natural Spa & Bath Oil*. Afterward, massage *T36-C7* into scalp and hair to soften and dislodge nits. Don't be stingy with the oil! Comb the oil through the hair. To fumigate the live insects, wrap your hair in a hot moist towel for 10 minutes. Repeat every second day for at least 5 treatments (10 days). Avoid re-infection. Wash all clothing and bedding with *MelaPower* laundry detergent and hot water.

BODY ODOR

Bacteria, yeast, bowel putrefaction, dental disease, vaginitis, chronic tonsillitis, kidney or liver failure as well as a number of chronic degenerative disorders and chemical exposures can lead to a foul body odor. Perfume was invented in Europe during the Dark Ages when the prevailing theory was that bathing and exposing the body to the air was the cause of infectious disease. WRONG! However, it may prevent people from getting close enough to you to give you a disease. Foul smelling sweat (bromhyperhidrosis) is observed in some diabetics, nervous individuals, chronic smokers and persons on certain prescription medications. People who have a bad odor become desensitized to it and need to be told by someone who cares. For more information, call *HEALTH TALK* and consult topics 29, 31, 44 and 46. Also, read the sections on Bathing, Sauna Bath, and Yeast Infections in this book.

TREATMENT: Drink 2 to 4 cups of *G'Day Melaleuca Tea* each day. Take *The Vitality Pak* regularly. Brush regularly with *Tooth Polish*, floss with *Dental Tape with T36-C7* and use *Breath-Away* Mouthwash after meals. Use *Hot Shot Mouth & Throat Spray* before going out in public. If you are a smoker, STOP! Bathe instead of shower. Use *Antibacterial Liquid Soap* and *Gold Bar* lavishly. Use *Defend Deodorant* after bathing and frequently during warm weather. Women can use *Nature's Cleanse* douche weekly. Pass the *"odor test"* from someone in your family before you use perfumes and colognes. When serious health concerns are causing the body odor, consult your physician. Take *ProVex* or *ProVex-Plus* daily.

BOILS

Raised, red, hard, hot and extremely painful pus-filled skin abscesses are caused by *Staphlococcus* organisms. They can appear anywhere on the body. Ears, nose, fingers and scalp are the most painful sites due to thin skin and constant pressure. The *Staphylococcus* organism may be contracted from farm animals and it can remain dormant in the body for years before erupting, usually when the person is run down, tired and over stressed.

TREATMENT: (NOTE: *Staphylococcus* **is very infectious and many strains are becoming resistant to prescription antibiotics.) Apply** *T36- C7* **every hour to a developing boil. Some boils can be stopped at this stage. Leave exposed to the air if possible. When a focal head begins to appear, usually after a couple of days, use a sterilized needle to lance the boil and allow drainage. The release of pressure usually provides immediate relief of pain. Continue applying** *T36-C7* **as long as drainage lasts. If possible, soaking the site in a solution of 1 oz** *Sol-U-Mel* **and 2 Tbs. Epsom salts in a quart of hot water can speed drainage. Then apply** *Triple Antibiotic Ointment* **to a soft gauze bandage and cover. Drink 2 to 6 cups of** *G'Day Melaleuca Tea* **each day. Take** *The Vitality Pak* **with every meal. If redness and swelling does not disappear after 7 days, see your natural physician. Take** *ProVex* **or** *ProVex-Plus* **daily.**

BRONCHITIS

Irritated bronchial membranes in the lung can swell and restrict air flow resulting in a condition known as bronchitis. Chronic cases can lead to asthma. Possible irritants include: low grade bacterial, yeast or viral infections, allergies, household cleaning chemicals, and irritation from cigarette smoke. For more information, call *HEALTH TALK* and consult topics 37, 38, 49 and 96. See the sections on Asthma, Chest Congestion and Coughing in this book.

TREATMENT: Treat the cause. Protect your air quality! Take *The Vitality Pak* daily. Drink 2 to 6 cups of *G'Day Melaleuca Tea* each day. Breathe the enriched steam from a vaporizer or a bowl of steaming water each morning and night before bed. To do this, add 5 drops of *T36-C7* to the water or receptacle in front of the steam jet. Form a tent over your head and the vaporizer or bowl, breathing the aromatic vapors through your nose and mouth gently into your lungs. Keep your eyes closed. Add 1 or 2 drops of *T36-C7* every 5 minutes for 15 to 20 minutes. For acute attacks, put 1 or 2 drops of *T36-C7* on a cotton tipped applicator and swab the inside of each nostril. (NOTE: Do not use *Sol-U-Mel* for the vaporizer treatment as it can cause irritation to the lungs.)

BRUISES

Ruptured blood vessels near the surface of the skin or in muscles can occur from injury, infection, or blood disorders. Discoloration is at first red, then black and blue, and finally green as healing takes place.

TREATMENT: The immediate application of ice to a traumatized area helps reduce bruising. *Pain-A-Trate* has a deep penetrating effect and reduces swelling, increases circulation, and speeds healing. Apply as often as needed until pain, discoloration and swelling disappear. If the bruise injury is near the eye, use caution to not get the oil in or too near the eye. Take *ProVex* or *ProVex-Plus* daily.

BUNIONS

Bunions are caused by the swelling of the second synovial joint bursa producing enlargement and displacement of the big toe which eventually laps over the second toe. They are sometimes caused by misalignment in the spine, causing improper biomechanics in the foot. Some cases have been linked to improperly fitted shoes during childhood development. Also, see on the section on Bursitis in this book.

TREATMENT: Apply *T36-C7* or *Pain-A-Trate* generously to the affected joint as often as discomfort exists. Soak in a solution of 1 oz *Sol-U-Mel* and 2 Tbs. of Epsom salts per quart of hot water each night. See your local chiropractor and ask for a walking gait analysis.

BURNS

No burn is simple to treat! This is true for a first degree burn which is red and swollen, a second degree burn which produces a blister, or a third degree burn which penetrates into muscle and deep tissue and occasionally chars the flesh. Infections, scars, and even shock can result if burns are improperly treated. Too much sun tanning damages skin cells. Ozone depletion in our atmosphere is increasing the amount of harmful ultraviolet rays from sunlight we are exposed to. There is an increase in melanoma skin cancer in those who are exposed to excessive ultraviolet radiation. Always protect your skin from sun exposure by using *Sun-Shades Sport Waterproof Sunblock SPF 15* if you have dark skin, or *Sun-Shades Max Waterproof Sunshield SPF 30* if you have a fair complexion.

TREATMENT: Immediately flush a fresh burn with cold water or apply ice and continue until the area is numb. Pat dry and apply *T36-C7*. Then cover with a thin coat of *Problem Skin Lotion*. Take *ProVex* or *ProVex-Plus* daily. Drink 3 to 6 cups of *G'Day Melaleuca Tea* per day. Most first degree burns will subside very soon. Repeat the *T36-C7* and *Problem Skin Lotion* application every hour until pain is gone. For second degree burns apply *T36-C7* and *Pain-A-Trate* immediately to prevent blistering. Repeat application of *T36-C7* and *Pain-A-Trate* each hour until pain and swelling is gone. Third degree burns require professional care, since deep blood vessels, nerves and lymphatic vessels in the skin are damaged. After cold application, apply *T36-C7* and *Problem Skin Lotion* or *Triple Antibiotic Ointment.* Cover with a sterile covering (the inside pages of an unused newspaper are sterile if other material is unavailable). Contact your doctor immediately. Skin grafting may be necessary. See the sections on Disinfectants and Antiseptics in this book.

BURSITIS

Small fluid-filled shock absorbing sacs are present in some joints such as the elbow, knee, shoulder, hip, ankle or great toe. Inflammation of these sacs, called bursa, causes swelling and painful movement of the joint. Trauma, infections, allergies or toxic accumulation are the usual causes. Gradual development from repetitive motion occupations can lead to chronic bursitis. Reducing coffee drinking curiously reduces bursitis of the shoulder. Acute bursitis can result from prescription drug reactions or sudden injury to the area. See the sections on Bunions and Gout in this book.

TREATMENT: Drink 2 to 6 cups of *G'Day Melaleuca Tea* per day. Take *The Vitality Pak* regularly. Take *ProVex* or *ProVex-Plus* daily. Apply *Pain-A-Trate* generously to the affected area every 2 to 4 hours. Moist heat may be helpful. Do not exercise the joint until pain and swelling is reduced.

CALLUSES

Thickening of normal skin caused by friction, usually on the hands or feet is seen in people whose work causes repeated pressure on a particular area. Brick layers, musicians, runners and surfers develop typical calluses. See the sections on Corns and Warts in this book.

TREATMENT: Minimizing the development of calluses is achieved by eliminating undue pressure to the affected site. Wearing softer and better fitting shoes, a moleskin or foam rubber protective bandage or arch inserts often helps.

Mela-Gel and *Problem Skin Lotion* applied before and after the activity helps to prevent friction at the active site.

CANCER PREVENTION

The second most common life threatening condition in North America is cancer. Almost one of every three citizens will develop cancer. Most will die from it in spite of the best care available. Prevention is still the wisest strategy. While no clear cause for all cancers is known, there appears to be a combination of circumstances that greatly increase the risk of cancer.

$$\text{Cancer Risk} = \begin{array}{lll} \text{Hereditary Tendency} & + & \text{Carcinogen Exposure} \\ \text{Immune Weakness} & + & \text{Time} \end{array}$$

By the same token, the formula for cancer prevention is practical and sensible which excludes it from scientific investigation and ridicule. Each one of us is responsible for our own health. Applying these simple facts to our life can give us the advantage we need. Here is the formula which many scientists agree is reasonable for preventing this dreaded disease as well as most chronic degenerative illnesses.

$$\text{Cancer Prevention} = \begin{array}{lll} \text{Optimum Diet} & + & \text{Exercise \& Rest} \\ \text{Positive Attitude} & + & \text{Lifetime Practice} \end{array}$$

TREATMENT: Whether or not you have had cancer, the recommendations included here can give you a greater measure of future cancer prevention. Many cancer researchers now believe that a combination of approaches to prevent cancer will prove to be the best treatment. Study your family tree for patterns of specific cancer types. Breast, colorectal, skin, prostate, uterus and lung cancers seem to be more hereditary linked. Tobacco (cigarettes, pipe, smokeless tobacco), fatty diet (animal or cooked vegetable oils), toxic chemical exposure (food additives, pesticides, herbicides, household cleaners, etc.), electromagnetic radiation (x-rays, TV, ultraviolet, etc.) and putrefying food in our digestive tract are the greatest known risks.

Get annual wellness checkups from a preventive physician. New blood tests (**PSA** for prostate, etc.) are being developed to detect antigens (immune sensitive chemicals) given off by early forms of cancer. Also, have a *Vitality For Life Personal Health Risk Appraisal* performed regularly to get a clear picture of your risks. Log your results from this report in the Health Appraisal Log in the appendix of this book for future reference.

Eat as if your life depended upon it, because it does! Take *The Vitality Pak* to ensure adequate anti-oxidants, B vitamins, and essential trace minerals, all of which are to some extent associated with cancer prevention. Take *ProVex* or *ProVex-Plus* daily. Drink plenty of pure water and *G'Day Melaleuca Tea* to continually detoxify. Apply *T36-C7* immediately to any suspicious skin lesion, mole, wart, skin tag or discoloration. Continue application 2 to 4 times each day until it disappears or until seen by your natural physician. Laugh, sing and play at least 30 minutes each day. Don't let the politics of treating cancer get in the way of your preventive program. Further information is found in my educational video tape on Cancer.

CANKER SORES

Mouth ulcers, known as canker sores, form on the gums and the inside of the cheeks. They are a localized bacterial infection characterized by a white scab appearance with a bright red border. The sores may be from pin head size up to the size of a dime, and are very painful. They can originate from a number of causes such as damage from brushing your teeth, biting your cheek, wearing dentures, or eating hard foods. Food allergies are often linked to repeated outbreaks. See the section on Cold Sores in this book.

TREATMENT: We have found that brushing with *Tooth Polish* and rinsing with *Breath-Away* reduces the bacterial count in the mouth. At the first sign of a canker sore, apply *T36-C7* to the injured site. Repeat every 4 hours.

CARDIOVASCULAR DISEASE

In 1912, the first case of atherosclerosis was documented in an elderly man. It was called a disease of old age and was a novelty which took up only one paragraph of a medical textbook. By 1960, cardiovascular diseases were the number one cause of adult death in North America. The war in southeast Asia identified 19 year old American soldiers killed in action who showed moderate to advanced plugging of the arteries in their hearts. In 1992, 485,000 Americans died from this disease. Researchers now suspect that dietary excesses and a sedentary existence may be the greatest contributors. What has happened to a people who are the envy of the world? We lack very little when compared to the rest of the world. Every president since John Kennedy has encouraged fitness proficiency in school children. Disease such as diabetes and high LDL cholesterol as well as smoking and eating a diet low in roughage and containing over 30 percent fat seems to be the pattern of most of those affected. A personal plan for prevention is needed by everyone. See the sections on Exercise and Cholesterol in this book. Further information is found in my educational video tapes on Healthy Hearts, and Stress.

TREATMENT: Prevention is the best treatment for cardiovascular disease. Stop smoking and avoid smokers. Have a *Vitality For Life Personal Health Risk Appraisal* performed regularly, and correct the risk factors in your lifestyle. Log your results in the Personal Evaluation Log in the Appendix of this book. Exercise regularly and eat an *Access Bar* 15 minutes before exercising to activate stored fat reserves for burning. Drink enough water and use *Sustain Drink* as a healthy snack alternative and meal replacement if you need to loose a few pounds of fat. Take *ProVex* or *ProVex-Plus* daily. Take *The Vitality Pak* with every meal to supplement your diet.

CARPAL TUNNEL SYNDROME

Those who use their hands with a continual repetitive motion, such as typists, experience a thickening of the nerve sheath in their wrists causing numbness, coldness and often pain. Any irritation

45

from the spinal cord to the hand can accelerate the problem. Prevention is the best line of defense. B-vitamins and trace minerals are needed, and specific wrist exercises often help. For more information, call *HEALTH TALK* and consult topic 56.

TREATMENT: First, eliminate the repetitive motion that caused the problem. Take *The Vitality Pak* with every meal until healing is completed (often 4 to 12 weeks). Apply *Pain-A-Trate* to the inside of the wrist and outside of the elbow every 4 hours to reduce inflammation and control pain. Avoid cold water. Hot water gives temporary relief.

CATARACTS

Damage from ultraviolet (UV) light, pollution or steroid drugs can lead to cataracts. Free radical damage causes clouding of the lens of the eye, slowly producing fuzzy vision and a halo appearance to lights at night. Surgical treatment is more successful in the young and healthy. Nutrition and alternative therapy provide hope for many who are not able to have the surgery. Prevention is the best treatment.

TREATMENT: Approved UV protective lenses should be worn by everyone who is exposed to sunlight or computer monitors. Avoid animal fats, antacids, and excessive sugar. Take *The Vitality Pak* and *Cell Wise Anti-Oxidants* with each meal. *ProVex-Plus* should be taken for both the treatment and prevention of cataracts.

CAT SCRATCHES

Scratches from all animals, including man, promote infection. Cat scratches are among the worst, because of the high population of bacteria growing on their claws. See the section on Disinfectants in this book.

TREATMENT: Immediately wash area with *Antibacterial Liquid Soap* or *Gold Bar*. Apply a few drops of *Sol-U-Mel* to the wet wash cloth for additional disinfection. Apply straight

T36-C7 to deep and bleeding wounds to speed drying and slow bleeding. Apply *Triple Antibiotic Ointment* to a sterile bandage and cover. Take *ProVex* or *ProVex-Plus* daily.

CHAPPED LIPS

Wind and cold takes its toll on mucous membranes of the lips. Fevers, medications and certain health conditions that lead to dehydration often cause chapped lips.

TREATMENT: Cracking and pain can be prevented and restored to normal within 1 to 12 hours by applying Melaleuca Lip Balm every 15 to 30 minutes. *Mela-Gel* can also be used to speed recovery.

CHEST CONGESTION

Reactions to viruses, dust, allergies, mold spores and physical activity can cause an accumulation of fluid, phlegm or mucous in the lungs and bronchial tubes. For more information, call *HEALTH TALK* and consult topics 35, 37, 38, and 49. Also read the section on Asthma in this book.

TREATMENT: Infections, including pneumonia, must be prevented. Irritations to the lung can rapidly develop into life threatening conditions. Breathe the vapor from 5 drops of *T36-C7* added to a warm steam vaporizer or a bowl of steaming water. For the best results, make a tent with a towel over your head. *T36-C7* or *Pain-A-Trate* can be applied to the chest to loosen congestion. Drink adequate amounts of clear liquids including *G'Day Melaleuca Tea* and broth. Avoid mucous forming foods such as dairy products, sugar and wheat. If congestion exists, use *CounterAct*, 1 tablet 3-4 times per day.

CHEST PAINS

Chest pains can be quite harmless or quite dangerous depending upon the cause. Emotional stress can cause chest tightness and localized pain. Air pollution can cause lung irritation and related chest pains. Persons who eat late in the evening, overeat, or eat in a hurry tend to have frequent indigestion and experience chest pains due to a hiatus hernia. This condition occurs when the stomach pushes up through the diaphragm due to gas in the bowel. On the other hand, when chest pain is from an occluded blood vessel, a reflex pain is usually felt extending from the chest into the left shoulder and neck area. A thorough checkup including a resting electocardiogram is recommended for active persons over 40 in an annual physical exam. Don't procrastinate! In over half of the cases of heart disease, there are no warning signs. A massive heart attack and death may be the only signs a doctor sees. For more information, call *HEALTH TALK* and consult topics 48 and 49. You may wish to see my educational video tape on Healthy Hearts.

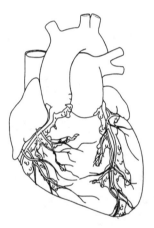

TREATMENT: See your natural physician if you have any chest pains! Listen to your body! Otherwise, have a *Vitality For Life Personal Health Risk Appraisal* performed. Slow down when eating and eat smaller portions. Decrease your dietary fat to 20% of your total calories. Begin a progressive exercise program to maximize circulation and oxygen to the diaphragm and heart. Minimize your sugar intake, as it is directly converted into fat within your body if you do not exercise enough. Maximize your lean body mass through weight training. Make sure you eat 2 fruit servings and 5 vegetable servings every day. Take *The Vitality Pak* daily to insure adequate nutrient levels.

CHICKEN POX

Chicken pox is a common contagious disease of children. The incubation period is usually 14 to 21 days. The symptoms start with a skin rash. Often a fever, headache and aching muscles are experienced. The rash changes into pimples and then blisters that enlarge and become filled with pus. The skin can become very itchy. Care should be taken to not scratch the affected areas to prevent scarring. The blisters dry up in a few days and are covered with scales. After all the blisters have scabbed, the disease is no longer contagious. For more information, call *HEALTH TALK* and consult topics 20, 21 and 88.

TREATMENT: Chickenpox is treated best by applying *T36-C7* directly on the vesicles. After the rash has fully developed, usually within 2 or 3 days, soaking in 1 oz of *Sol-U-Mel* and 1 oz of *Natural Spa & Bath Oil* in a tub of warm water for 15 minutes can help the itching. Drink one to four cups of *G'Day Melaleuca Tea* daily.

CHIGGERS

Walking through the grass in the Summer in the Mid West and the South occasionally results in painful, itching eruptions on the feet, legs and thighs. The female mite digs into the flesh and lays eggs that cause a sore. The larva hatch and then bore under the skin causing an intense dermatitis. For more information, call *HEALTH TALK* and consult topics 19 and 20. Also read the section on Scabies in this book.

TREATMENT: Rub *T36-C7* on the area of the bites each morning and evening. Follow by applying *Triple Antibiotic Ointment* to prevent secondary infection. Large areas can be treated by soaking in a warm tub with 1 oz of *Sol-U-Mel* and 1 oz of *Natural Spa & Bath Oil* while scrubbing with a wash cloth and *Antibacterial Liquid Soap*. For prevention, apply *T36-C7* to the bottom of pant cuffs or spray pants and socks with 1 oz *Sol-U-Mel* diluted with 7 oz of water.

CHOLESTEROL

This naturally occurring starting material for many hormones has been misunderstood mainly because of half truths published in the news. Here is the other half of the story. There is *good* cholesterol (made from balanced nutrition during exercise and play) and *bad* cholesterol (made during stress or over-cooked animal fats). Cholesterol is needed for life. It is our body's own anti-oxidant protecting us against naturally occurring free radicals. We need a certain amount of cholesterol to handle stress. We make about four times as much cholesterol in a day as we eat in our diet. Excess dietary fat (including margarine) tends to increase blood cholesterol. People who have high blood cholesterol and high stress cannot lower blood cholesterol by avoiding it in their diet. Adequate fiber and roughage in the diet carries fat and toxic substances quickly out of the body. Heat converts normal cholesterol found in animal products into oxycholesterol which is unhealthy and toxic. The original heart disease scientists in the 1970's told us about the dangers of too much cholesterol in our blood. Today the researchers are telling us about the dangers of it being too low! Further information is found in my educational video tape on Circulation.

TREATMENT: Have a *Vitality For Life Personal Health Risk Appraisal* performed and begin following the recommendations for reducing risk factors. Take *ProVex* or *ProVex-Plus* daily. Take *The Vitality Pak* supplements with each meal. Begin a regular exercise program and eat an *Access Bar* 15 minutes before your work out. Put *Sustain Drink* in your water (1 tbs. per quart) while working out to maintain needed energy and electrolytes. Drink 2 to 4 cups of *G'Day Melaleuca Tea* each day.

CIGARETTE SMOKING

Imagine a 747 jumbo jet filled with passengers crashing every hour of every day within the United States borders. How long would this tragedy be allowed to continue? Of all the plagues of man, cigarette smoking has probably caused more deaths and resulted in more disease than all other non-infectious causes combined. Over 50 toxic or banned substances have been identified resulting from smoking; including carbon monoxide, carbon dioxide, dioxane, arsenics oxide, biphenyls, and cadmium salts just to name a few. Nicotine, after the Latin name of the plant meaning nightshade, is a powerful insect repellant, aphid killer on roses and deadly poison which will not be eaten by animals in the wild. Smoking one cigarette reduces the infection fighting ability of the immune system by 50 percent for 2 hours. It has been advised against by the March Of Dimes since 1974 for causing birth defects. Second hand smoke has been linked to a 15% lower IQ among children of households where at least one parent is a smoker. Nicotine is an addictive alkaloid drug related to codeine, morphine and cocaine. Recently, cigarette companies have been accused of actually adding nicotine to their higher priced brands to induce greater addiction and desire for their product. Many congressmen list financial holdings in the lucrative tobacco industry which may account for the 30 year struggle to gain governmental bans of this deadly waste of human health. Further information is found in my educational video tape on Detoxification.

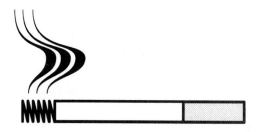

TREATMENT: There is no greater single health measure you can take than to quit smoking and forbid the practice in your home or around your loved ones. Like any drug addiction, it must be faced with courage and compassion. If you have the personal strength to stop smoking - do it right now! If you need help, seek a natural physician who is trained in chemical addiction treatment with diet, herbs, acupuncture and hypnosis. Take the *Vitality For Life Personal Health Risk Appraisal* and begin a lifestyle of wellness rather than self destruction. Take *ProVex* or *ProVex-Plus* daily. Take *The Vitality Pak* every meal. Drink 2 to 4 cups of *G'Day Melaleuca Tea* each day.

51

COLD SORES

Very painful clear, fluid filled eruptions of the border of the mouth, forming hard, oozing scabs resulting from an infection of either the herpes simplex or herpes facialis virus. Once thought to be more common in infants and children, adults are becoming more susceptible. The infection makes chewing difficult and may impede the appetite. Mild damage associated with exposure to the sun, stress, abrasions from a toothbrush, bad allergies to certain foods, the onset of menstruation, or any disease that produces a fever or increases metabolic rate may produce a lesion. As a rule, the symptoms generally go away after 7 to 10 days. Dehydration and secondary infections give reason for concern.

TREATMENT: Since the virus feeds on an excessive intake of the amino acid Arginine, diets avoiding citrus fruit and nuts should be followed. Supplementation with the amino acid L-Lysine, found in most health food stores, is advised to stop the early spread of the infection. Dab *T36-C7* on the lesions immediately upon detection. Repeat every hour until the lesion either disappears or comes to a head. The former is the typical case. If it comes to a head, continue to apply *T36-C7* once every 2 hours followed by *Mela-Gel* or *Problem Skin Lotion*. For persistent or large surface sores, use *Triple Antibiotic Ointment* every 4 hours.

COLIC

Chronic severe abdominal pain can be caused from a number of conditions which may be non life threatening. See the section on Appendicitis in this book. Newborns may experience colic when the digestive system has not developed enough to handle food properly. Gas or constipation is the usual cause of the abdominal pain. Heavy metal poisoning (lead, copper, zinc, cadmium, etc.), food or environmental allergies, ovarian cysts, gallstones, kidney stones, intestinal parasites, pesticide residue from produce, food poisoning, chlorine poisoning and chronic constipation can all cause colic. For more information, call *HEALTH TALK* and consult topic 94.

TREATMENT: Get a thorough examination from your natural physician to identify the cause, if possible. A hot moist pack with *Pain-A-Trate* on the affected area gives some relief. Soak fruits and vegetables in 2 quarts of cold water and 1/2 tsp. of *Sol-U-Mel* for 10 minutes then rinse in pure water. Detoxify by using only steamed and juiced vegetables at least one meal each day. Drink 1 to 2 quarts of water, plus 2 to 4 cups of *G'Day Melaleuca Tea* per day. Take the *This Is Fiber?* bars as a snack. Exercise regularly.

For the infant suffering from colic, there are several treatments to consider. The food source is the first possible problem. Mother's milk is best for an infant, at least for the first four months. If colic is present, the mother may need to be careful not to eat any rich, spicy, or gas forming foods. Also, if she is experiencing stress, her milk may be affected. So stay calm and get plenty of rest. Do not introduce any other foods for the baby until advised by a natural physician. If the baby is drinking formula, he may be having an allergic food reaction. A change in formula may be needed. Gas is a common cause of colic. Gently but firmly patting the baby on his back or bottom should help eliminate the gas. Giving the baby a pacifier may help reduce tension and colic. If constipation is a serious concern, a physician will suggest some possible solutions for the baby.

COMMON COLD

Cold viruses attack the moist, cooler regions of the nose, throat, sinuses, vocal cords, and larynx when our systems are run down. The virus has developed a way of avoiding destruction by the immune system and is present in a dormant state. Apparently, when we contact a cold from someone else, (sneeze, handshake, kiss) the two viruses exchange fragments of genetic information to form a slightly new strain. It is new enough to enter living cells undetected where it begins to multiply until cell damage has taken place and the immune system drives the virus into seclusion until the next opportune time arises. Mucous membranes become swollen, red and irritated as the virus spreads from one cell to the next. Untreated colds can progress into more threatening conditions.

TREATMENT: The common cold usually gives a warning that it is about to develop. From the earliest signs of tiredness, sneezing and hoarseness you are given a few hours to launch an attack. Immediately take a hot bath (See the section on Bathing in this book). Also, breathe the steamy vapor of *T36-C7* for 15 minutes (air temperatures above 104 degrees kill the virus - that is why we get the chills and then a fever, so speed up the fever). See the section on Chest Congestion in this book for directions for steam vapor treatment. Apply one drop of *T36-C7* to each nostril of your nose every 4 hours. Sip vegetable broth and/or mom's chicken soup every couple of hours. Avoid any temptation to eat solid foods as your digestive tract, including smell and taste, are on vacation for awhile. Try a hot *Sustain Drink* to fight any fever you may produce. Take *MELA-CAL* 4 times a day to reduce painful muscles. *"Drown the cold"* with *G'Day Melaleuca Tea*, 1 cup per hour. Get all the rest you can. If you start early, you can beat it in 24 hours, otherwise, it will take a week or more for the virus to run its course. If congestion exists, use *CounterAct*, 1 tablet 3-4 times per day.

COMPRESSION FRACTURES

Automobile accidents, athletic injuries, falls, chronic muscle spasms and decreased bone calcium (See Osteoporosis) can cause the vertebrae of the spine to squeeze together with sufficient force to break the bone. After the age of 25, very little blood circulation is available to properly heal the injury. For more information, call *HEALTH TALK* and consult topic 55.

TREATMENT: See your physician for professional care. Diagnosis of compression fractures requires an x-ray. Take *MELA-CAL* 3 to 6 times per day to minimize pain from muscle spasms. Apply *Pain-A-Trate* to the affected muscles and gently, but firmly, massage above and below the affected area. Take *ProVex* or *ProVex-Plus* daily.

CONJUNCTIVITIS

An irritation of the pink skin flap of the eyelid can be caused by a bacterial infection (often contagious), allergy (itching and burning) or chemical contact (red and painful). Children often get contagious *"pink eye"* from playmates. Consult your natural physician. For more information, call *HEALTH TALK* and consult topic 23.

TREATMENT: I have had good success treating mild conjunctivitis in the early stage by putting 5 drops of *T36-C7* in a warm steam vaporizer and slowly blinking the eyes carefully in the direct path of the vapor. Repeat every 5 minutes for three consecutive doses before bed. Repeat morning and night for 3 days. If the irritation persists, see your natural physician. Take *ProVex* or *ProVex-Plus* daily. Note: Do not put any *Melaleuca* products directly on the eye. Use only products that are certified ophthalmological grade.

CONSTIPATION

It is healthy and normal to have a bowel movement within one to two hours after eating. Wastes, including undigested fiber, pass out of the healthy body within 12 hours after eating the meal. Poor diet, lack of exercise, not drinking enough water, stress, and many drugs can cause constipation. We are a constipated society. Colorectal diseases are at an epidemic level. See the section on Hemorrhoids in this book. Further information is found in my educational video tape on Colon Health.

TREATMENT: I have found four things that help most sufferers of constipation: Eat enough fiber; Drink enough liquids; Get enough exercise to maintain bowel mobility; and Don't worry so much. Specifically, get 20 to 30 grams of fiber each day. (Note: 1 medium apple + 1/2 cup of old fashioned oatmeal + 1/4 cup raisins + 2 carrots + 1 cup of

broccoli + 1/2 cup of cooked beans = 10 grams of fiber).
Take the *This Is Fiber?* Bars to maximize fiber. Drink 1 to 3
quarts of water including *G'Day Melaleuca Tea* each day.
Take *ProVex* or *ProVex-Plus* daily. Run, walk, jog, bike or
swim, etc. for 30 minutes each day. Replace thoughts of
fear or worry with happy, optimistic thoughts. This releases
hormones in the bowel which aid digestive juices and
propel food along the bowel and out of the body.

CORAL CUTS

While skin diving in Hawaii a number of years ago, I learned
first hand how dangerous swimming around coral can be. I
attempted to take a short-cut cross the jagged coral reef. As the surf
tossed me around like a cork in a washing machine, I developed cuts
and gashes whose scars have left a vivid memory of the event. A
doctor friend irrigated the wounds, disinfected them with trusty
Melaleuca alternifolia oil, and sutured my legs, belly and elbows.
He said that some people swell up like a balloon from infection one
or two days after coral cuts. Prolific microbes live in sea water and
on the saber spines of coral. See the section on Disinfectants in this
book.

TREATMENT: The cuts are often jagged and irregular and
harbor bacteria which necessitates thorough cleansing with
pure water and *Antibacterial Liquid Soap* enriched with
Sol-U-Mel. Remove particles of sand and coral. Apply *T36-
C7* or *T40-C5* for maximum disinfection. Suturing wounds
which cut through the skin and into muscle, speeds healing
and reduces secondary infection. Apply the *Triple
Antibiotic Ointment* over the stitches, if applicable, and
cover with a gauze bandage. Daily inspect the wound for
redness or swelling, which gives indication of the spread of
infection. Soak feet and hands in a solution of 1 oz *Sol-U-
Mel*, plus 1 oz of *Natural Spa & Bath Oil* plus 1/4 cup
Epsom salt in 1 quart of hot water. Rinse open wounds
daily with 1 oz of *Sol-U-Mel* in 1 pint of water. Change the
dressing daily and reapply *Triple Antibiotic Ointment* or
Mela-Gel.

CORNS

Corns are raised areas of hyperkeratosis or thick callus skin which are caused by friction or pressure often over a bony extension of the foot, such as the ball of the foot or the toe joints. Corns are first noticed as pea size or slightly larger and occur on the side and bottom of the feet. Hard corns occur over the toes and soft corns occur between the toes. Corns may ache spontaneously or become very tender upon pressure. Proper fitting shoes will help prevent corns. See the section on Calluses in this book.

TREATMENT: Soak feet in a solution of 1 oz *Sol-U-Mel* and 1 oz of *Natural Spa & Bath Oil* in 1 quart of hot water for 15 minutes. Proceed twice daily until the corn softens enough to remove the core with tweezers. Apply *Triple Antibiotic Ointment* or *Mela-Gel* and cover with a small bandage.

COUGHING

Our bodies produce phlegm and mucous in the throat and lungs when exposed to severe temperature changes, chemical irritation or allergens. We instinctively cough to remove this phlegm and foreign substances. Smoking is the most common cause of chronic coughs. See the section on Smoking in this book. Severe coughing can cause bleeding of the throat or inner ear infections. For more information, call *HEALTH TALK* and consult topics 35 and 36.

TREATMENT: Treat the cause - Eliminate your exposure to the irritating substances. In mild cases, breathe the vapor of 5 drops of *T36-C7* in a bowl of steaming water for 15 minutes while holding your head over the bowl. Make a tent over your head and the bowl with a bath towel. Repeat morning and evening. Drink the *G'Day Melaleuca Tea* throughout the day. If congestion exists, use *CounterAct*, 1 tablet 3-4 times per day.

CRAMPS

Sudden decreases in tissue oxygen, in muscle or nerve calcium levels, or hormonal changes before menstrual flow can trigger muscle cramps. Side aches during or after strenuous exercise are due to diaphragm spasms caused from low oxygen and low calcium levels in that muscle.

TREATMENT: After eating a meal, wait 45 minutes before exercising. Properly stretch and warm muscles before exercise. *MELA-CAL* taken 4 times per day and at bedtime can prevent sub-optimum levels of calcium in the blood and prevent cramps. Eat an *Access Bar* 15 minutes before exercise. Drink *Sustain Drink* during and immediately after exercise. A warm bath and a good massage can help reduce pain greatly. Massage *Pain-A-Trate* into muscles which cramp easily.

CUTICLES

The rolled skin at the edge of the finger and toe nails can give evidence of your general health. Dry cuticles which split and become infected, are often due to exposure to harsh soaps or solvents such as gasoline or paint thinner. See the section on Dry Skin in this book.

TREATMENT: After washing hands with *Antibacterial Liquid Soap* or the *Gold Bar*, apply *Hand Creme* to the hands and work into the cuticles to prevent dryness. Apply *Triple Antibiotic Ointment* or *Mela-Gel* to infected cuticles. If condition persists, see your natural physician.

CUTS

If the object that caused the injury was dirty or exposed to disease causing organisms, extra care must be taken in thorough cleaning. Cuts should be treated soon after injury. If you work around animals or farm equipment, or work in a food handling industry, make sure your tetanus shots are current.

TREATMENT: Clean the affected area with a wash cloth, warm water, and Antibiotic Liquid Soap and/or *Sol-U-Mel.* Apply *T36-C7* and keep clean with a bandage. Check the healing progress daily. Re-clean and apply new bandages as often as needed. Deep or wide cuts may require a visit to your natural physician for suturing.

DANDRUFF

This dry flaking of the scalp is one of the most common conditions affecting the adult population. White, scaly skin sloughs off of the head in a *"snow storm"* fashion to disgrace the victim. The use of poor quality soaps and shampoos can irritate the sebaceous (oil) glands and produce a dry scalp that flakes off when combing or brushing. The condition upsets the normal healthy skin bacteria and adds to the unsightly condition the typical itch. Because of our chemical and perfumed countenance, dandruff proliferates.

TREATMENT: Avoid harsh soaps, shampoos, or hair care products. Shampoo with *Natural Shampoo* or *Herbal Shampoo.*

DEAFNESS

Gradual loss of hearing in adults can be due to the incurable condition of nerve loss caused from viruses, infections, high fevers, prescription drugs, and trauma. One estimate is that 20 percent of the adult population is hearing impaired. Partial hearing loss can often be helped with hearing aids. Some adults go through the best years of their lives never knowing what they are missing.

Over one half of the adults we examine have accumulated wax in one or both ears, which impedes hearing to some extent. Ear wax cleaning is an important preventive practice for small children as well as adults. Some reoccurring middle ear infections in children permanently disappear when the ears are kept clean. Some people need their ears cleaned as often as once or twice a year.

TREATMENT: To remove excess ear wax that may be interfering with hearing, follow the treatment directions in the section on Ear Wax in this book. Get a hearing test from a qualified audiologist.

DECAYED TEETH

Dentists have done an admirable job in helping prevent tooth decay. Brushing, flossing and swishing after eating has become a way of life for most of us. None-the-less, some decay still takes place. Dentists and scientists argue that the use of fluoride, while definitely reducing tooth decay in some, may pose a greater risk in the long run to the general health of the body.

Refined foods (mainly sugar in its many forms) promote rapid yeast, bacterial and other micro-organism growth in the many cracks and crevices in and around the teeth. (You would not believe how many frightening creatures I have removed from the mouth and showed patients with my dark field microscope.) These microbes secrete acids which erode the calcium rich enamel of the teeth. Proper brushing and flossing habits are essential to reduce the microbial population. See the section on Baby Teeth in this book.

TREATMENT: Gently brush the teeth and tongue after every meal. Swish mouth with *Breath-Away* to reduce mouth microbes as well as to control jungle breath. Floss frequently. Have regular checkups with your dentist to maintain healthy teeth.

DERMATITIS

Inflammation of the skin with redness, oozing, crusting, scaling and sometimes vesicles can be sudden and short lived or chronic in nature. More than 50 percent of all skin conditions I see in my practice can be classified as dermatitis. Chronic dermatitis is commonly known as eczema.

Healthy skin is able to withstand exposure to many natural substances and some synthetic chemicals without harmful effects (it is designed to be our first line of defense against the outside world). Substances which irritate the skin include plants such as poison ivy, some trees, some fruits and vegetables, therapeutic drugs such as cortisone and antibiotic creams, cosmetics and hair dyes, fabrics such as wool and synthetics, as well as toxic household cleaners and chemicals. In addition to these external sources there are internal conditions such as allergies and sensitivities to foods and prescription and over-the-counter drugs that often cause dermatitis. Further information is found in my educational video tape on Skin Care.

TREATMENT: Identify the cause of the dermatitis before aggressively treating the symptoms. As soon as possible after the symptoms begin, wash the area with *Antibacterial Liquid Soap* or *Gold Bar*. Additional soaking in a warm tub with 1 oz of *Sol-U-Mel* and 1 oz of *Natural Spa & Bath Oil* is advised.

DIABETES

Juvenile onset diabetes appears to be due to a defective gene that causes self-destruction of insulin producing cells in the pancreas. Insulin must be taken regularly to support life. Adult onset diabetes, on the other hand, appears to be due to suppression or inhibition of normal pancreas production. Being over 55 years of age, overweight, lack of exercise, high refined sugar consumption and dietary fat consumption of more than 20% of daily calories is the typical picture. Usually, insulin is unnecessary but a pancreatic stimulant drug is often prescribed. For more information, call *HEALTH TALK* and consult topic 1. You may wish to see my educational video tape on Diabetes.

TREATMENT: With either type of diabetes, have a *Vitality For Life Personal Health Risk Appraisal* performed and follow the advice. Drink 2 to 4 cups of *G'Day Melaleuca Tea* each day and take *The Vitality Pak* with each meal. Take *ProVex* or *ProVex-Plus* daily. Make exercise and low fat, low sugar eating a way of life.

DIAPER RASH

Common diaper rash is caused by friction and irritation in the presence of moisture, which triggers yeast to grow. This occurs naturally when wet diapers are not changed promptly. Hospital nurseries often harbor resistant strains of these organisms. You may bring them home with your new bundle of joy. Elderly or incontinent adults must also beware of this problem.

TREATMENT: Properly launder all baby clothing as well as diapers in hot water enriched with 1 oz of *Sol-U-Mel* per load. *Sol-U-Mel* should be used sparingly, if at all, in bath water as the green soap in it may irritate sensitive skin (newborn babies lack active sweat glands). *Natural Shampoo, Antibacterial Liquid Soap* or *Gold Bar* should be used to bathe your baby. After towel drying your baby, allow skin to air dry (in direct sunlight if possible) for a few minutes. Apply *Triple Antibiotic Ointment, Body Satin Lotion* or *Hand Creme* to form a natural moisture barrier on the skin before diapering.

DIARRHEA

A sudden increase in stool volume, fluidity, or frequency of fecal excretion is seen with microbial infections, flu viruses, stress, food poisoning, laxatives, certain genetic and malabsorption problems, and electrolyte loss from vomiting or drugs. The greatest concern is depletion of body fluid resulting in vascular collapse (the heart has nothing to pump). Children under the age of 4 can dehydrate quickly and die from uncontrolled diarrhea.

TREATMENT: NOTE: Determine the cause, if possible. If there is abdominal pain, fever, or if the diarrhea does not resolve rapidly, seek emergency help without delay. Otherwise, begin drinking *G'Day Melaleuca Tea*, 4 to 16 oz every hour along with *Sustain Drink* for energy and nutrient replacement.

DISINFECTANTS

Selectively reducing the population of disease-causing germs to make room for the friendly germs, without harming humans or household plants and animals, is what a good disinfectant does. Sanitation engineers have taught us that in order to control the spread of disease, we must control the number and transportability of disease causing germs. Several products are effective and especially stand out for their use in making safe play-toys, furniture, clothing and bodies. See the Appendix in the back of this book for a comparison of the disinfectant properties of *T36-C7* compared to other agents.

TREATMENT: Sponge bathe a sick person with *Antibacterial Liquid Soap* or *Gold Bar* on a wash cloth to reduce surface germs often transported through perspiration. Disinfect the air by running a warm steam vaporizer with *T36-C7* in the sick room. (See Air Purification) A general disinfectant solution for a sick room is a solution of 1 oz *MelaPower* laundry detergent plus 1 oz *Sol-U-Mel* in 1 gallon of warm water. Sponge, mop or wipe floors, walls, door knobs, lamps, bed frames.

DIVERTICULOSIS

Chronic constipation, insufficient fluid intake, inadequate dietary roughage, and some medications can cause pressure in the lower bowel sufficient to cause bulges or sacs in the muscular wall. These bulging pockets, or diverticuli, can become impacted with fecal material and extend to over one inch in length. If improperly cared for, they can develop irritation, pain and serious infections, a condition known as diverticulosis.

TREATMENT: Until about 20 years ago, a low roughage diet was recommended for treating diverticulosis. Puddings, white bread, Jell-O and soft vegetables proved however, to do little to stop the surgeon's knife. Oat bran, wheat bran, and psyllium, along with adequate exercise and liquids is my treatment of choice for diverticulosis. Adequate roughage found in *This Is Fiber?* and *G'Day Melaleuca Tea*, 2 to 4 cups per day, is a good way to increase bowel elimination and reduce pressure. *The Vitality Pak* is needed for healing and improved health.

DIZZINESS

Most of us have experienced motion sickness when we whirl around, ride a merry-go-round or go out on the ocean in a small boat. The feeling that objects are moving around us tricks our equilibrium mechanism in the inner ear and can even be due to an optical illusion (Omni Vision). Several health conditions can make us susceptible to this feeling such as middle ear infections, tumors, toxicity from drugs or alcohol, brain injuries and concussions. One of the most common causes of unexplained dizziness is from low blood sugar in reactive hypoglycemia or after exercise. Diabetics can get it from insulin reactions.

TREATMENT: See your natural health doctor if unexplained dizziness is occurring. For blood sugar control, I recommend that small meals be eaten often throughout the day instead of large meals eaten less often. Avoid sugary foods, since this causes sudden drops in blood glucose from the rebounding insulin release. Take *The Vitality Pak* supplements daily. Eat an *Access Bar* 15 minutes before exercise so your body can burn fats instead of running out of fuel. If you get dizzy easily during or after exercise, drink *Sustain Drink* in your water while working out.

DRUG POISONING

Three out of every ten hospital admissions are due to either prescription or over the counter drug reactions. Sixteen hundred people die each year from aspirin poisoning alone. Be certain that your drug oriented doctor communicates all possible side effects from any needed medications. Eli Lily, pharmacist and founder of Lily Pharmaceuticals is quoted as saying, *"A drug without side effects - is no drug at all."* Dermatitis, nausea, accelerated heart rate, excessive sweating, stomach pains, and diarrhea are some of the milder reactions. Tumors, kidney failure, diabetes, ulcers and sudden death are the more common severe reactions. One pharmacist friend of mine says that only one third of prescriptions are taken in the proper dosage or for the duration that they are prescribed. Other authorities state that the overuse of prescription antibiotics has resulted in super resistant strains of bacteria which defy all known treatment and killed over 13,000 hospitalized patients in 1992 alone. Some drugs react with others to produce baffling symptoms. When several doctors are treating the same patient for different conditions, the risk of drug interactions increases. The most recent Physicians Desk Reference lists over 2300 reactions from drugs - many from misuse. Be informed and realize that the majority of drugs are for *"treating symptoms"* only and do not offer a cure! If your doctor says you will need to take the drug for the rest of your life, he or she is often referring to this philosophy. Only the body can cure! Prevention and common sense can reduce the need for many drugs and their potential side effects on us and our environment.

TREATMENT: Always ask you medical doctor or pharmacist to list the possible side effects of the prescription drugs you are asked to take. Drink *G'Day Melaleuca Tea* every hour to speed detoxification. Take *ProVex* or *ProVex-Plus* daily to help detoxification.

DRY SKIN

Some people have dry skin due to hormonal or nutrient deficiencies, prescription medications or a deficiency of essential fatty acids in their diet. Hands that work in caustic or cold environments or those that are washed frequently (food handlers or health care workers) will develop excessively dry cracked skin. Women who are going through the change of life are very prone to dry skin and chapped hands. The decreased production of natural oils reduces moisture in skin.

TREATMENT: Wash in *Antibacterial Liquid Soap* then apply *Problem Skin Lotion* liberally. Apply *Triple Antibiotic Ointment* or *Mela-Gel* to cracked or infected areas. *Hand Creme* can be used on hands after washing to help restore moisture. When hand chapping has begun, apply *Problem Skin Lotion* every 4 hours until normal skin moisture is restored. Skin dryness which has invaded deeper tissues, or caused swelling will require treatment with *Triple Antibiotic Ointment* every 4 hours, to control infection until healing is accomplished. *Pain-A-Trate* has been used by some patients with poor circulation. Take *The Vitality Pak* with each meal.

EAR INFECTIONS

Repeated ear infections with fever and pain (See Earaches) requiring cycles of antibiotics are a sign of continual blockage of the ear canal. Infections of the outer ear (pinna) can travel into the ear canal where severe pain is produced. Permanent hearing loss or meningitis can result if treatment is delayed. If antibiotics are unsuccessful, the use of tiny Teflon tubes are often surgically inserted through the eardrum, which allows accumulating fluid and pus to drain outward from the ear. The tubes are occasionally expelled within a few days or weeks and constitute a major part of some pediatricians practice. Other pediatricians refuse to use this technique because of questionable results and the rare chance that they may travel deeper into the middle ear to create new problems. Swimmers, bottle-fed infants and recently immunized children frequently populate my waiting room with ear infections.

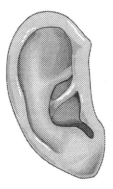

TREATMENT: Don't overlook allergies as a cause of repeated ear infections. Identify the cause, if possible. See your natural physician if in doubt. Never send a child outdoors with an ear infection. To treat an ear infection, a drop of warm *T36-C7* or *T40-C5* can be applied full strength or mixed with 5 to 10 drops of olive oil or other neutral oil to saturate the end of a cotton plug. This is inserted in the outside ear canal and left over night. Avoid using full strength *T36-C7* in children's or sensitive adults ears as local irritation can result. The vasodilation (local warming) effect is therapeutic, but should be diluted first to not produce further pain. A hot water bottle or heating pad set on low should be put over the ear. Drink 4 to 16 ounces of *G'Day Melaleuca Tea* every hour to prevent dehydration from the fever. If congestion exists, use *CounterAct*, 1 tablet 3-4 times per day.

EAR WAX

Some people produce more ear wax than others. Some people also produce hard wax while others make soft ear wax. There is some relationship between excessive ear wax production and high blood lipids (cholesterol or triglycerides). Ear wax may plug the ear canal and cause itching, pain, and temporary hearing loss.

TREATMENT: To clean excess or impacted wax from the ear canal, do the following. Apply one drop of *T36-C7* and one drop of *Sol-U-Mel* to a small piece of cotton which has been pulled and twisted to a point. Insert the soaked point in the ear canal overnight. The next morning, remove the cotton and fill a rubber baby syringe (purchased at any drug store) with a solution of 1 tsp. *Sol-U-Mel* in 8 ounces of water heated to body temperature. Hold the syringe toward the side of the canal just inside the ear opening, leaving a space for the water to swish back out. Squeeze a firm stream of water into the ear canal several times to melt and dislodge the wax. NOTE: Old wax may require the application of a heating pad to the ear for about 10 minutes before irrigating. If the wax is too hard or too large, consult your natural physician.

EARACHES

Unlike adults, the ear canal in infants and small children inclines upward from the inner ear toward its exit in the throat. This anatomical uphill climb makes children more susceptible to earaches and inner ear infections. You do not have to have infection to have earaches. Milk drinking after weaning, allergies, the common cold, and even teething can cause this problem. Symptomatic relief is often given with antihistamines, aspirin and Tylenol. A cool breeze can set off ear canal muscle spasms. I have removed many foreign substances from children's ear canals including beans, beads, blueberries, a live moth (very painful), and rocks. Using cotton tipped swabs to clean the ears can push wax and other materials to the back of the ear canal against the ear drum causing damage. Rapid changes in air pressure (such as landing in an airplane) quickly identify the children and adults who have Eustachian tube congestion. For more information, call *HEALTH TALK* and consult topic 25.

TREATMENT: **Note: Determine the cause of the pain, if possible. Cover a child's ears when out in cold or windy weather to prevent earaches. Loose cotton pushed into the outer ear canal can help protect sensitive ears. Holding the open end of Styrofoam cups firmly over the ears when landing an airplane has a dramatic effect on preventing earaches in adults as well as children. A drop of warm *T36-C7* or *T40-C5* can be mixed with 5 to 10 drops of olive oil or other neutral oil to saturate the end of a cotton plug. This inserted in the outside ear canal and left over night will help minimize pain. Avoid using straight oil in sensitive ears as local irritation can result. I used full strength oil with our daughter but had to dilute the oil to 1:10 with our son. Diluted warm *T36-C7* can be dripped into an ear that has a live bug inside. This will kill the bug so it can be removed painlessly. If congestion exists, use *CounterAct*, 1 tablet 3-4 times per day.**

EDEMA

Hot weather, lack of exercise, kidney, liver, or heart problems as well as drug toxicity can cause swelling due to excessive sodium and water retention. Sudden weight gain of 2 to 15 pounds in a few days may be the first signal. Obesity, fatty diet, salty foods, carbonated beverages, and excessive sugar tend to increase edema. Lower legs, ankles and feet are the most often affected. Facial puffiness usually denotes kidney disease. One way to test for edema is to press on the inside of the ankle with moderate finger pressure. If a *"pit"* is seen when pressure is released, this means there is excessive fluid trapped in the space between cells. Edema that develops only toward the end of the day most often responds to diet, exercise and stress control. For more information, call *HEALTH TALK* and consult topic 61.

TREATMENT: Have a *Vitality For Life Personal Health Risk Appraisal* performed and begin following the suggestions. Exercise regularly. Drink 2 to 6 cups of Melaleuca Tea each day and take *The Vitality Pak* with each meal. Elevate the legs for 15 minutes in the mid-afternoon and evening. Wear support hose when standing or walking for prolonged periods.

EMPHYSEMA

Mature adults who have been exposed to air pollutants or who have smoked develop this illness. The germ and pollution digesting enzymes that are released by the white blood cells cause permanent damage to the tiny air sacs in the lung. The person has trouble exhaling and develops an enlarged or over extended chest. A simple spirometry test (lung volume) and history usually tells a story of hard work and an abused life. If the person also has allergies, further development of asthma is common. See the sections on Air Purification, Asthma, and Bronchitis in this book.

TREATMENT: Treatment to prevent further damage includes stopping smoking, getting moderate exercise unless the heart is also damaged, drinking 2 to 4 cups of *G'Day Melaleuca Tea* daily, and taking *The Vitality Pak* with each meal. Steam inhalation each night with a few drops of *T36-C7* is helpful to prevent infections from bacteria, yeast and fungus. Follow the directions under the section on Bronchitis in this book. If congestion exists, use *CounterAct*, 1 tablet 3-4 times per day.

EXERCISE

Why should we exercise? Because we are designed to be physical creatures as well as emotional and spiritual. A better word for this activity is play! Children expend more daily calories per kilogram of their body weight than adults because of their attitude about play. The purpose of exercise is to improve the efficiency of combining oxygen with fuel to produce energy. In the clinical laboratory this is measured as the $VO_{2\ max}$, (maximum volume of oxygen used per unit time). The word *aerobics* (done with oxygen) describes exercises that tend to improve or condition the body to do this more efficiently. In order to achieve the greatest benefit, an exercise must be chosen which is enjoyable, comfortable and ideally performed at a level of exertion that a casual conversation can be maintained. Physically exhausting activities should be avoided if better health is the goal. Having an exercise target helps to get the most from your activity. Your target heart rate is based on an equation developed by exercise scientists. You must have a watch with a second hand and be able to take your pulse in your wrist or feel it in your neck.

220 - Your Age x 0.8 = Your Target Heart Rate

Example: if you are 50 years old

220 - 50 x 0.8 = 136 beats/minute
(about 14 beats in 6 seconds)

This is 80% of your maximum attainable heart rate (at 100%, your heart is put under too much stress). Exercise helps to reduce the resting heart rate. The most complete body exercises are swimming, jumping on a trampoline, and cross country skiing, because they use so many muscles. The next best exercises are walking, hiking, jogging, soccer, bicycling, aerobic dancing and skating. Court sports such as tennis, racquetball, handball, basketball and volleyball are good, but do not keep the heart rate even enough to sustain the conditioning effect. Other activities usually need to be included in your weekly work out schedule if you want better overall health. Weight lifting, bowling, archery, baseball, and horseback riding are more anaerobic (done without oxygen) and are great sports, but cannot provide the kind of activity to keep the blood and oxygen adequately supplied to all organs of the body. Always make sure that you have adequate hydration before you start to exercise. (I drink 1 quart of liquid before each daily work out.)

70

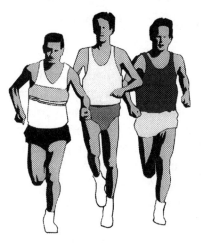

TREATMENT: Take *Vitality Pak* with each meal. Eat an *Access Bar* 15 minutes before exercise. Drink *Sustain Drink* throughout and after exercise.

EXERCISE STRAIN

There are several levels of muscle strain. Mild strain occurs regularly with all forms of exercise. Severe muscle strains can cause tearing and bruising. See the section on Bruises in this book.

TREATMENT: Overused muscles, tendons (connecting muscles to bones), and ligaments (connecting bones to other bones) are helped by immediately applying ice to prevent swelling. Keep the ice on for 5 to 10 minutes each hour, until the swelling is reduced. *Pain-A-Trate* gives dramatic relief from athletic strains. I carry *Pain-A-Trate* in my racquetball bag and use it often on ankles, calve muscles, knees, wrists, elbows and low back areas before pain sets in. It is wonderful used this way.

EYE INJURIES

Never put *T36-C7*, *Triple Antibiotic Ointment*, or *Mela-Gel* in the eye as they can cause pain and dryness of the eyeball. None of the medicine chest products are approved for use in the eye. For more information, call *HEALTH TALK* and consult topic 23. Also read the section on Bruises in this book.

TREATMENT: If the injury is due to caustic chemicals splashing in the eye, you should immediately wash the eye with fresh water for several minutes. Contact your eye doctor without delay. Foreign matter in the eye can scratch or even penetrate the cornea. Avoid rubbing the eyes, so as not to cause further irritation. Note: Do not put any *Melaleuca* products directly on the eye. Use only products that are certified ophthalmological grade.

FATIGUE

Fatigue is the second most common complaint doctors hear. Fatigue is more than tiredness; it is an inner feeling of difficulty in performing the most basic physical tasks and usually leads to a *"bad attitude"*. It can be caused from serious disorders such as anemia, cancer, chronic viral infections, low thyroid hormone production, hypoglycemia, diabetes, allergies, premenstrual syndrome, and the near-exhaustion phase of stress or emotional crisis. It can also be due to correctable factors such as inadequate sleep, malnutrition or habitual sedentary lifestyle. Clinical depression is often associated with fatigue. Consult the sections on Allergic Reactions and Anemia in this book. For more information, call *HEALTH TALK* and consult topic 66.

TREATMENT: Have a *Vitality For Life Personal Health Risk Appraisal* performed and begin following the recommendations. Balance exercise with rest. Identify and avoid possible allergic foods in your diet.

FEVER

A rise in body temperature to 100.4 degrees (2 degrees above normal - the new normal temp is 98.4) is considered a fever. A portion of the brain known as the hypothalamus measures the temperature of the blood. It stimulates hormones to increase the rate of burning fuel and directs blood flow away from the skin, causing chills. In this way, the body has its own internal thermostat. Bacteria and viruses give off hormone-like substances, known as pyrogens, which trigger the same body reaction. A fever that comes and goes or lasts over two weeks may involve the *"resetting"* of the hypothalamus to a higher temperature. Certain types of cancer and brain tumors can cause this. Scientists now generally agree that a fever, up to a point, is healthy and is the body's attempt to *"burn"* the foreign substance or organism out of the body. For more information, call *HEALTH TALK* and consult topics 5, 89, 93.

TREATMENT: If a fever is less than 103 degrees, drink liquids, including G'Day Melaleuca Tea, every 1 to 2 hours and restrict activity. Since fevers tend to reduce appetite, restrict solid food. If a fever is above 103, a tepid (warm to normal skin - about 99 degrees) enema is helpful to bring the temperature down. If the fever is above 105 for more than 2 or 3 hours, emergency measures should be taken to reduce it and prevent brain damage.

FOOD POISONING

Bacteria can spoil improperly cared for food. Bacterial wastes called exotoxins trigger fever, chills, nausea, stomach and muscle aches, diarrhea, headaches, and dizziness. Many people come down with the *"flu"* after eating a picnic lunch on a hot summer day. *"Traveler's Flu"* usually affects entire families. Improperly canned low acid foods, such as green beans, can grow botulism producing organisms which are fatal! Shellfish, chicken, chemical food additives, mushrooms, and reheated leftovers are common causes of food poisoning.

TREATMENT: When traveling, prevention is assured by eating in restaurants which have a reputation for safety. Avoid foods from street vendors. When in an area where the quality of food is unknown, eat only fruit that can be peeled and avoid raw vegetables and salads made from raw vegetables. Care must also be taken, especially in hot weather, to keep perishables cold. As soon as food poisoning is suspected, induce vomiting to minimize absorption of bacterial exotoxins. Drinking a half cup of

warm water containing one teaspoon of salt usually works. If possible, drink one cup of boiled *G'Day Melaleuca Tea* every hour. *This Is Fiber?* should be eaten every few hours to speed bowel transit and hold toxins in the stool. If vomiting or diarrhea persists, dehydration is a concern. Obtain medical care if this condition lasts for more than two days in an adult, or one day in a child.

FOUL TASTE IN MOUTH

The human taste buds are highly developed in some people. Certain food tastes are pleasant to some and not so pleasant to others. Disorders of taste can be caused from sinus infections, reduction in smell due to nasal congestion, smoking, or facial nerve damage. Other conditions causing foul tastes are poor dental hygiene, chemical poisoning, heavy metal poisoning, viral infections or psychological depression. Reduced taste can be due to zinc deficiency in the diet.

TREATMENT: If organic causes for the foul taste cannot be determined, begin a systematic treatment plan of your own. Proper daily dental care with *Tooth Polish, Breath-Away* Mouthwash and *Hot Shot Mouth & Throat Spray* can be very helpful in restoring normal taste. Have regular dental checkups. Take *The Vitality Pak* with each meal. Drink 2 to 4 cups of *G'Day Melaleuca Tea* each day. Avoid being around pesticides and herbicides as well as solvents, paints or petroleum based products. If you experience frequent nasal congestion, consult your natural physician for allergy testing.

FROSTBITE

Exposure to freezing temperatures can cause ice crystals to form in and between cells, which causes cell damage. The skin stings, itches, burns, and sometimes turns red and/or numb. Peeling or blistering may occur in 24 to 72 hours. Lifetime sensitivity to temperature may develop.

TREATMENT: Frostbite can usually be prevented by protecting the body with warm, dry clothing, paying close attention to the hands and feet. When frostbite is suspected, immediate action must be taken to warm the affected area. Since numbness can be an advanced symptom, care should be taken to not overheat the area. Soaking for 30 minutes in water 100 to 110 degrees Fahrenheit is advisable. Then apply *Pain-A-Trate* to maintain micro-circulation. Repeat the soaking and application of *Pain-A-Trate* every hour for four hours. The affected body part can become sensitive to cold after one attack and can easily suffer other attacks. Regular exercise and massage can help improve circulation in the area.

FUNGAL INFECTIONS

Several considerations are involved in understanding fungi. These organisms belong to the plant kingdom and are found on all healthy skin. Many infections are caused by opportunistic forms of fungi that take advantage of a person's weakened immune system. As such, fungal infections are common in people receiving x-ray therapy, taking birth control drugs, steroids, or antibiotics, diabetics, burn victims, and people with TB or emphysema. Many infections develop during tropical vacations or military service. Severity can vary from a mild rash on the skin, to a fatal overgrowth in the lungs. When the infection is localized, it is more easily treated than if it has invaded a major organ. Because of the many forms of fungal infections, microscopic examination of the affected tissue, hair shaft, or sputum is helpful in making a diagnosis. Fungal infections fail to respond to antibiotics and can successfully be treated with Melaleuca oil. Fungal infections have different names depending on the area of the body affected:

Skin (*Tinea corporis*)	-	See Ringworm
Feet (*Tinea pedis*)	-	See Athlete's Foot
Nails (*Tinea ungium*)	-	See Ringworm
Scalp (*Tinea capitis*)	-	See Ringworm
Groin (*Tinea cruris*)	-	See Jock Itch
Beard Area (*Tinea barbae*)	-	See Barber's Itch

GALLSTONES

Excessive dietary fats, high cholesterol, habitual weight loss diets, drugs that effect the liver, a family history of gallstones, birth control pills, and excessive dietary sugar most commonly are associated with gallstone formation. Dull upper back pain, especially near the right shoulder blade, after eating a fatty meal is the most common symptom of gallstone formation. Sudden nausea with pain in the upper mid or right stomach area heralds a gallbladder attack, usually at night after retiring. Chemical analysis of blood and stool samples can determine if conditions for gallstone formation are present.

TREATMENT: Prevention is best! Have a *Vitality For Life Personal Health Risk Appraisal* performed and begin following the recommendations. Avoid fatty foods, and reduce dietary fat intake to less than 20% of the total calories each day. Eat *This Is Fiber?* Bars to keep bile flowing through the bowel. Avoid sugar and sugar containing foods.

GANGRENE

Caused by bacteria, gangrene is a progressive infection that causes death to the tissues and if untreated, will require amputation. If caused by the clostridium bacteria, moist gangrene causes blisters, oozing fluid, and putrid odors, thus the term gas gangrene. It also has the symptoms of dry gangrene where the affected area turns black, looses feeling and has red inflamed surrounding tissue. Some of the causes of gangrene are bad wounds and infections, reduced blood supply to an extremity, diabetes, frostbite, drug reactions, and swelling from large burns. Warning symptoms include pain in the area when at rest, and black, blue, or purple colored skin around the affected area. See the sections on Disinfectants, Diabetes, and Frostbite in this book.

TREATMENT: See your natural physician if symptoms are suspicious. Depending upon the location and advanced state of the infection, antibiotic therapy may be ineffective and often fails to stop the disease. If caught in the early stages, soak the body part in a solution of 1 oz of *Sol-U-Mel* and 4 Tbs. Epsom salts in one gallon of very warm water (106 to 110 degrees) for 20 minutes every 2 hours. The wound should be allowed to drain as much as possible. Keep the area warm, since the tissue usually feels hot and swollen. Apply *T36-C7* or *T40-C5* every 2 hours to the affected part. *Pain-A-Trate* can increase local blood circulation to the area and should be applied immediately after *T36-C7* or *T40-C5*.

Gastric Ulcers

Stress, aspirin, or spinal nerve irritation as well as a poor diet, can lead to ulcers by stimulating the Vagus nerve, which controls production of stomach hydrochloric acid. Some scientists insist that the taking of antacids, while giving temporary relief from stomach acid, in the long run actually elevates production of stomach acid. Statistics show that while antacids are being taken at ever increasing frequency, ulcers continue to be one of the most frequently treated conditions. Starting as indigestion and stomach pain, this condition can lead to referred back pain, anemia and fatigue if uncorrected. Our high-stress lifestyle appears to be the most contributing factor. For more information, call *HEALTH TALK* and consult topics 41 and 42. You may wish to see my educational video tape on Liver and Gall Bladder.

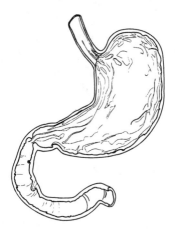

TREATMENT: For persons having ulcers for several years or more, lifestyle should be closely evaluated. Along with your doctor's directions, have a *Vitality For Life Personal Health Risk Appraisal* performed and follow the advice. Drink 2 to 4 cups of *G'Day Melaleuca Tea* each day. Begin an exercise program. Practice relaxation breaks for 20 minutes each day. For acute attacks, drink one cup of *G'Day Melaleuca Tea* every hour. Eat one half of a *This Is Fiber?* bar every 2 hours between meals. Eat cole slaw or have boiled cabbage every four hours (compound U in cabbage stops production of stomach acid). Avoid alcohol, caffeine, smoking, and rich or fatty foods, as these stimulate the production of stomach acid.

GASTRITIS

Gastritis is an irritation in the stomach and/or small intestine, usually caused by gas. Overeating, eating in a hurry, or eating rich foods late at night are the usual causes. Severe gastritis can trigger pains in the chest which are often mistaken for a heart attack. Further information is found in my educational video tape on Digestion.

TREATMENT: Celebrate eating by giving thanks, having soft music and candle light. Take time between bites to have casual conversation, and quit eating just before you are full. If gastritis is common, in spite of these preventive measures, avoid eating anything 3 hours before bedtime, and avoid drinking anything within 1 hour of bedtime. Drink liquids only between meals including *G'Day Melaleuca Tea*. Persistent discomfort should be brought to the attention of your natural physician.

GLOSSITIS

Inflammation of the tongue is a sign of a local irritation, or more often, a disease elsewhere. Local causes can include mechanical trauma from jagged teeth, ill-fitting dentures, or repeated biting during convulsive seizures. Other irritants include alcohol, tobacco, hot foods, and spices, or sensitization to chemicals in toothpaste, mouthwashes, breath fresheners, candy dyes or dental materials. The most common general cause of glossitis is malnutrition or avitaminosis (a deficiency in specific B vitamins). A few rare disorders produce tongue inflammation but are determined by first ruling out these common causes. For more information, call *HEALTH TALK* and consult topic 29.

TREATMENT: Take *The Vitality Pak* every meal. Stop smoking. Use only safe dental hygiene products such as *Tooth Polish, Breath-Away* and *Dental Tape with T36-C7*. Drink 2 to 4 cups of *G'Day Melaleuca Tea* per day. Have dental checkups regularly. If congestion exists, use *CounterAct*, 1 tablet 3-4 times per day.

GOUT

Painful joints of the toes, fingers, or other areas, along with elevated blood uric acid is typically known as gout. Sharp urate crystals cause physical damage to the cartilage. Persons eating rich animal products, those getting high percentage of calories from cereal grains (gluten converts to urates in some people) and excessive fruit sugar (fructose stimulates urate production) are known to suffer with this condition. Once known as a *"rich man's disease"*, gout affects those who over-indulge in such conveniences as pizza, hot dogs, and high fructose corn sweetener laden beverages. Vegetarians have been alarmed to discover the cause of their pain was grain and fruit induced gout.

A related condition known as pseudogout (similar symptoms, but without elevated blood uric acid) is due to calcification of cartilage in the affected joint. X-rays usually indicate the presence of pseudogout and it is occasionally associated with dairy product sensitivity or toxic drug reactions. For more information, call *HEALTH TALK* and consult topic 62.

TREATMENT: Have a *Vitality For Life Personal Health Risk Appraisal* performed and begin following the recommendations. Start a low stress diet consisting of more vegetables (a *"greens and beans diet"*) and fewer animal products. Drink the 2 to 4 cups of *G'Day Melaleuca Tea* each day. Apply *Pain-A-Trate* to any affected joints 2 to 4

times each day at first, then each morning and evening until painless mobility is achieved. Hot soak with 1 capful *Sol-U-Mel* in 1 quart of water 30 minutes each morning to minimize damage to cartilage.

HAIR LOSS

One cause of hair loss can be an inherited trait seen in middle aged men. A receding hair line is caused by an accumulation of male hormones, which alters the natural fats secreted in the scalp and stunts hair growth. The characteristic pattern is thinning and baldness beginning in the front and progressing backward over the head. Research has recently shown that men who begin this pattern in their 20's or early 30's instead of the mid-forties have a greater risk of developing heart disease early in life. Male pattern baldness or slow hair loss due to aging has no known proven treatment. It appears to be nature's conservative desire to reduce unneeded plumage as we get older! We do know that protein metabolism (hair is pure protein) slows down by about one-half after the sixth decade of life. We also know that maximizing our nutrition in youth helps avoid or postpone many genetic weaknesses called inborn errors of metabolism.

In conditions other than male pattern baldness, we find quite an array of causes. I have seen partial hair loss in children who were malnourished, patched hair loss due to heavy metal poisoning such as lead, thinning or splitting and lifeless hair due to harsh chemical hair care products, total body hair loss due to stress and intermittent hair loss in persons experiencing bowel parasitic infections. After giving birth, some women will lose up to one-third of their head hair, but quickly grow it back within a year if properly nourished. I have even seen a few cases of head lice, and also dog and cat flea bites that have produced immune reactions in the scalp of children which causes temporary hair loss. Dandruff sufferers, due to scratching, often have mild to heavy hair loss. See the section on Dandruff in this book. Complicated or unresponsive hair loss should be evaluated by your natural physician.

TREATMENT: After ruling out the pathological conditions causing hair loss, I have seen a number of people slow down or stop hair loss when simple steps were taken. A

daily scalp massage with *T36-C7* or *Problem Skin Lotion* is often helpful. Use *Natural Shampoo* to maintain healthy hair and scalp. Above all else, get adequate nutrition including protein. Take *The Vitality Pak* with each meal. Adequate rest to prevent stress is essential. Include moderate exercise in your daily schedule to keep the pores of the skin clean and skin circulation optimal. Drink *G'Day Melaleuca Tea* on a daily basis.

HAY FEVER

Hay fever is one of the most commonly seen conditions. Its seasonal symptoms of tree, weed, and grass pollen hypersensitivity include runny, red and itching eyes and a runny stopped up nose. The victim may also experience sneezing, a loss of smell, a sinus infection, and the ears may be stopped up. See the section on Allergic Reactions in this book.

TREATMENT: When possible, avoid exposure to the pollens you are allergic to. Due to cross sensitivity, food allergies may reinforce pollen allergies. For example, eating wheat may aggravate a wheat pollen allergy. Avoid eating wheat, oats, rye and barley from May until August. Each night before retiring, swab each nostril of your nose with a cotton tipped applicator containing *Problem Skin Lotion*. This will reduce the accumulated pollen from the day and moisten dry mucous membranes. Take *The Vitality Pak* each meal to boost your immune system. Drink 2 to 4 cups of *G'Day Melaleuca Tea* each day. If congestion exists, use *CounterAct*, 1 tablet 3-4 times per day.

HEADACHE

There are many types, degrees of severity and locations of headaches. About 80% of all headaches are due to muscle tension or nerve restriction from stress or injury, which inhibits blood flow out of the brain. These respond well to chiropractic adjustment of the vertebral spine and massage of tense muscles. Allergies, eye strain, sinus or dental infections, viruses, high blood pressure, reduced blood oxygen, low blood sugar, or toxemia (constipation, alcohol, chemical fumes, caffeine addiction, etc.) are other common causes. Brain tumors can also cause slowly developing, continual headaches. Migraine headaches usually are one sided and can be severe enough to cause nausea and reduced vision. Migraine sufferers get dramatic relief from identifying and eliminating specific sensitized foods from their diet. For more information, call *HEALTH TALK* and consult topic 9.

TREATMENT: For tension headache, gentle massage for 2 to 5 minutes to the back of the neck, on the temples, on the sinuses over and under the eyes using *Pain-A-Trate* often relieves local muscles and promotes blood circulation. Take special care to keep *Pain-A-Trate* away from your eyes. Applying a hot moist pack to the back of the neck, temples, or over the eyes afterwards completes the treatment. Most tension headaches are relieved within 10 to 15 minutes with this technique. If symptoms do not improve, keep a log of the frequency, severity, and duration of your headaches and see your natural physician. Remember, do the simple things first! Have a *Vitality For Life Personal Health Risk Appraisal* performed and begin an exercise program to reduce tension. Take *The Vitality Pak* with every meal. Drink 2 to 4 cups of *G'Day Melaleuca Tea* each day. Take a *This Is Fiber?* bar to maximize bowel elimination. Take *Sustain Drink* between meals to maintain blood sugar. Drink water and get plenty of rest. If congestion exists, use *CounterAct*, 1 tablet 3-4 times per day.

HEART PALPITATIONS

Heart beats you are aware of are referred to as heart palpitations. They can be a normal response, such as occurs immediately following exercise or when excited. Severe physical stress, anxiety, or an over active thyroid are common causes of unnatural palpitations. Organic heart disease, such as clogged arteries, enlarged heart, congestive heart failure, or ischemia also cause heart palpitations. Some people notice skipped beats or extra beats of their heart. If a feeling of weakness, light-headedness or difficulty getting a breath accompanies palpitations, consult your physician without delay. See the section on Allergic Reactions in this book. For more information, call *HEALTH TALK* and consult topic 48.

TREATMENT: Reduce stress! Learn to relax! Have a *Vitality For Life Personal Health Risk Appraisal* performed and follow the advice supplied. Take *The Vitality Pak* at each meal. Drink 2 to 4 cups of *G'Day Melaleuca Tea* per day.

HEAT EXHAUSTION

Prolonged exposure to high temperatures may lead to either excessive fluid loss, gradual weakness, anxiety, nausea and excess sweating, or failure to sweat, headaches, weakness, and sudden loss of consciousness (heatstroke). Advanced cases of heat exhaustion are emergency situations, requiring immediate cooling of the body to prevent death. For more information, call *HEALTH TALK* and consult topics 5, 6, 89 and 93.

TREATMENT: Common sense is the best preventive measure. Strenuous exertion or wearing heavy, insulated clothing in a hot or inadequately ventilated environment should be avoided. Fluids and electrolytes should be replaced by drinking cool (not too cold) *G'Day Melaleuca Tea* or *Sustain Drink* every hour. If exposure to heat is prolonged for several days, and heavy perspiration is maintained, *The Vitality Pak* should be taken with every meal to replace lost minerals and maintain temperature regulation mechanisms within the brain. If conditions are severe, get immediate medical attention.

HEMORRHOIDS

Hemorrhoids are varicosities of the veins of the hemorrhoidal plexus in the anus, often accompanied by inflammation, reddening, and bleeding. Seldom are they painful unless accompanied by more advanced conditions such as fissures (tears) or fistulas (burrow-like tracts from the inner anus to non-healing sores around the anal area).

Over 50% of adults are bothered by hemorrhoids. There are biblical accounts of piles (hemorrhoids). Hemorrhoidal veins contain blood that is not emptying properly into the portal circulation to the liver. Constipation, laxative induced diarrhea, pregnancy, and occupations requiring long seating on hard or cold objects tend to cause this itching, burning irritation. Constipation causes excess lower bowel pressure and can cause the external hemorrhoid veins to enlarge suddenly. Thin or flat-on-one-sided stool or a full feeling immediately after a bowel movement is a good indication of internal hemorrhoids. For more information, call *HEALTH TALK* and consult topics 45-47.

TREATMENT: Preventing this condition is best. Get adequate exercise each day. Drink adequate fluids including 2 to 4 cups of *G'Day Melaleuca Tea* each day. Take *ProVex* or *ProVex-Plus* daily to promote healing. A *This Is Fiber?* bar should also be taken every day to prevent constipation. A cotton ball or 2 x 2 inch gauze pad soaked with *T36-C7* or *Pain-A-Trate* held in the anal opening can quickly reduce the itching and burning. Chronic hemorrhoids are best treated by adding 1 oz of *Sol-U-Mel* and 1 oz of *Natural Spa & Bath Oil* to 1 quart of warm water. Sponge the solution onto the hemorrhoidal area. Leave for several minutes. Pat dry. Apply *Problem Skin Lotion* or *Triple Antibiotic Ointment*. Repeat the procedure morning and night for seven days. A hot sitz bath each evening with the above solution may be very helpful in shrinking any external hemorrhoids. Stubborn hemorrhoids may require conservative therapy beyond the use of Melaleuca products. A treatment known as Keesey Electro-desication, which has been used for over 60 years, is very effective. There is very little discomfort with the treatment and the person is able to resume regular work activities right away. Contact your natural physician.

HICCUPS

These are repeated involuntary spasms of the diaphragm, followed by sudden closure of the glottis, which stops the inflow of air and produces the characteristic sounds. Some people are more prone to hiccups from drinking alcohol, taking certain medications, bladder irritations, excitement and certain disorders of the stomach, or bowel. High blood carbon dioxide seems to reduce hiccups.

TREATMENT: Many different treatments have been tried from the very simple (holding your breath) to quite extreme (surgically cutting the nerve going to the diaphragm!). The most common do-it-yourself methods that may work are: breathe in and out deeply but slowly into a paper bag (not plastic as it may cling to nostrils); take series of deep breaths and hold them as long as possible; swallow dry bread, honey or crushed ice; induce vomiting; pull and hold the tongue; put direct finger pressure on "your" eyeball; drink cool *G'Day Melaleuca Tea* from the far side of a glass by bending your head down between your knees. In spite of all these methods, including surgery and powerful drugs, some cases of hiccups have been recorded to last for weeks. Thank goodness, I have found the above conservative treatments quite effective. Good luck.

HIGH BLOOD PRESSURE

No single cause is known for hypertension. Whatever the cause or causes, it will lead to either a restriction of blood flow in the blood vessels or increased heart pumping. Family tendencies are often seen as the most common trait. Lifestyle factors such as type *"A"* personalities (high stress), smoking, high blood cholesterol and triglycerides, alcohol consumption, and caffeine consumption predominate. Contrary to popular belief, salt consumption in healthy people does not increase blood pressure. (Low blood pressure, however, is often due to a deficiency of salt) Persons who are under high stress and have high blood pressure benefit from restricting salt intake. Actually, deficiencies in many other essential nutrients including magnesium, potassium, and B vitamins are known to be present in people who have high blood pressure, and are helped by supplementation. See the section on Cardiovascular Disease in this book.

TREATMENT: Have a *Vitality For Life Personal Health Risk Appraisal* performed and follow the advice. Progressive exercise helps high blood pressure by reducing stress hormones and increasing the efficiency of the vascular system. Take *The Vitality Pak* with each meal. Take *ProVex* or *ProVex-Plus* daily to promote vascular integrity. Drink 2 to 4 cups of *G'Day Melaleuca Tea* each day.

HIVES

Hives are a form of skin rash that consists of raised white welts mixed with red patches on the skin. Drug allergies, severe stress, insect stings or bites, ingestion of certain foods (particularly eggs, shellfish, nuts or fruits), and desensitization injections can cause hives from a hypersensitive reaction. Certain virus infections such as hepatitis, mononucleosis and measles can be announced by the sudden appearance of hives. Hives lasting 2 weeks or longer can be due to an allergic reaction to drugs or chemicals such as penicillin in milk, non-prescription drugs, food preservatives, dyes, or other food additives. Hives can also result from animal dander. For more information, call *HEALTH TALK* and consult topics 18, 20 and 22.

TREATMENT: The cause of hives is an allergic or hypersensitive reaction. Determine the source and avoid it in the future. Application of *T36-C7*, Mela-Gel, *Pain-A-Trate,* or soaking in a warm bath with 4 oz of *Sol-U-Mel* and 4 oz of *Natural Spa & Bath Oil* usually returns normal circulation to the affected area. Drink *G'Day Melaleuca Tea* 2 to 4 times each day to assist detoxification. Chronic hives can be due to an underlying disease and should be brought to the attention to your natural physician. If congestion exists, use *CounterAct*, 1 tablet 3-4 times per day.

HOARSENESS

Hoarseness is due to inflammation of the voice box (larynx) and can be caused from simple overuse, such as yelling at an athletic event, or other disorders such as viral or bacterial infections. For more information, call *HEALTH TALK* and consult topic 34.

TREATMENT: Inhale steam made from a bowl of boiling water and 5 to 10 drops of *T36-C7*. Drink hot *G'Day Melaleuca Tea* 2 to 6 times each day. Resting the voice usually reduces the symptoms within a few days and prevents further inflammation.

HOT FLASHES

Not to be confused with a fever, hot flashes can appear suddenly with a stiflingly stuffy hot feeling and reddened sweaty head, face and neck skin lasting from a few seconds to several minutes. They are often followed by chills. Hot flashes occur in over 75% of women at menopause and may occur for more than 5 years. Pregnant women may also experience hot flashes. Apparently, the hypothalamus of the brain becomes unable to coordinate with other hormone fluctuations and body temperature changes, due to declining estrogen levels. Stress plays a moderate part. For more information, call *HEALTH TALK* and consult topic 6.

TREATMENT: Cell Wise contains antioxidants which help some women minimize hot flushes. Up to 6 or 8 tablets per day for at least one month, along with *The Vitality Pak* with each meal and drinking *G'Day Melaleuca Tea* is often effective. Daily exercise and stress reduction is important.

HOT TUBS

No Melaleuca products, including *T36-C7*, *Natural Spa & Bath Oil* or *Sol-U-Mel*, should be used in an operating hot tub or permanent Jacuzzi tub. *Melaleuca alternifolia* oil is not compatible with the filtration system in these sophisticated environments.

HYPOGLYCEMIA

Low blood sugar accounts for more behavioral symptoms than any single condition. Afternoon fatigue, forgetfulness, dull headaches, multiple food allergies, anti-social behavior, difficulty loosing weight, bad dreams, sweet or alcohol cravings, sudden loss of energy, eating disorders, fits of anger or depression, body aches, poor protein digestion and slow physical reflexes are the more common symptoms. Stress, over consumption of refined sugar, and nutritional deficiencies of minerals and B vitamins appear to be the causes of hypoglycemia. Up to 50% of Americans randomly tested with a 6 hour glucose/insulin tolerance test have an abnormal response. Since the nervous system cannot store fuel, it must constantly be bathed in glucose for normal function. (One judge in California is noted as not granting a divorce to couples until they have both taken a glucose tolerance test.) Children experiencing hyperactive behavior following a sugary holiday are well documented by teachers. In adults, sudden drops in blood sugar or low fasting levels (before breakfast) stimulate instincts to eat something or somebody! Many convicted criminals have a history of sugar abuse. Alcohol is the simplest form of sugar. Untreated hypoglycemia in some people, tends to produce adult type diabetes. For more information, call *HEALTH TALK* and consult topics 1, 3, 7-9, 12, 24, 42, 54, 55, 63-70.

TREATMENT: **Eat nourishing meals with the insurance of *The Vitality Pak*. Avoid refined sugar, caffeine and cooked fats. Exercise moderately after eating an *Access Bar*. Take *Sustain Drink* between meals to prevent sudden blood sugar drops.**

INCONTINENCE

Involuntary loss of urine during the day or night (bed wetting) occurs in the very young and very old, naturally. About 3% of children have a congenital defect of the urethra which causes leakage and often requires surgical repair. About 12% of the adult population experiences symptoms as mild as dribbling when laughing, sneezing, lifting or coughing; or it can be experienced by an urgent desire to void followed by involuntary loss of urine. Stress or urinary tract infections can be the possible cause. Mature men with an enlarged prostate gland can have urinary incontinence or retention. Whatever the cause, loss of control of the urinary sphincter muscles is the result. I have found back injuries, food allergies, alcoholism, emotional disturbances and B vitamin deficiencies to be causes of urinary incontinence. For more information, call *HEALTH TALK* and consult topics 53 and 98.

TREATMENT: A simple chiropractic low back adjustment for children who wet the bed may solve the problem. Other children in my practice were rid of this embarrassment only after they stopped drinking milk. Some needed a good B vitamin supplement added to their diet. *Vita-Bears* or *The Vitality Pak* should be taken with each meal. Women with urinary infections (less than half have any pain or discomfort) should drink 2 to 6 cups of *G'Day Melaleuca Tea* each day - earlier in the day is better. A series of pelvic tilts, called the Kegel Exercises, are helpful for women who loose urine when they laugh or cough. For those with a stressful lifestyle, have a *Vitality For Life Personal Health Risk Appraisal* performed and follow the advice for stress reduction and exercise. Men over the age of 40 should have a blood test called a PSA performed regularly. *The Vitality Pak* should be taken with each meal along with 2 to 6 cups of *G'Day Melaleuca Tea* to protect the prostate.

INDIGESTION

Gas, belching, or a bloated feeling is a sign of inadequate digestion in the stomach. Eating on the run, inadequate chewing, dilution of digestive juices with copious amounts of liquids, and stress all play a great part in causing indigestion. We now know that, in the long run, antacids can actually make the problem worse. Malabsorption, ulcers, constipation, and low bowel conditions including hemorrhoids and cancer are seen frequently in people who have a history of indigestion. See the sections on Gastric Ulcers & Constipation in this book. For more information, call HEALTH TALK and consult topics 41-44.

TREATMENT: Celebrate eating. Sit down. Give thanks. Surround yourself with people you love as often as you can. Savor each bite. Use just enough seasoning to bring out the natural taste. Take time to let the mystery of life begin the process of converting the protein, starches and essential oils into living flesh and blood. Take *The Vitality Pak* with each meal. Drink 2 to 4 cups of *G'Day Melaleuca*

Tea each day - between or after meals. For more serious digestive problems, consult your natural physician.

INFLUENZA

Influenza is an infectious disease caused by a virus. Its' many symptoms may include chills, fever, cough, headache, aches in the joints, weakness, and stomach distress. Much more severe than the common cold, the flu can progress to total exhaustion, acute bronchitis, pneumonia, and sometimes death. (The great flu epidemic of 1917 killed over one half million people.) Since the virus is spread from one person to another, controlling the environment is important. Keeping ones immune resistance up is the best prevention. See the sections on Air Purification, Disinfectants, and Fever in this book. For more information, call *HEALTH TALK* and consult topics 1, 5, 28, 33, 35 and 96.

TREATMENT: Upon the first signs of the flu, start drinking *G'Day Melaleuca Tea* and hot *Sustain Drink* to prevent exhaustion. Go to bed. Don't try to control the fever unless it gets over 104 in a child or 103 in an adult. Begin a steam vaporizer with *T36-C7* in the infected person's room. Apply *Pain-A-Trate* to strained neck and chest muscles. Take Cell Wise every 2 to 4 hours for the antioxidant effect which reduces pain of muscles, chest and abdomen.

INGROWN TOENAILS

Ingrown toenails are due to tight fitting shoes or the improper breaking-in of shoes. One method of preventing a recurrence is to file a V notch on the middle of the nail so that the point nearly touches the quick. This will cause the nail to draw towards the center and prevent the embedding of the edges of the nail. Trimming in a rounded fashion is not recommended as this actually causes further ingrown toenails.

TREATMENT: If possible, carefully remove the ingrown part of the nail. Soak the foot for 15 minutes in a solution of 1 oz *Sol-U-Mel* per quart of hot water. Dry thoroughly. Apply

T36-C7 followed by *Mela-Gel* or *Triple Antibiotic Ointment.* Repeat morning and night. If there is an infection, see the section on Abscesses in this book.

INSECT BITES

Most plagues and life threatening communicable diseases have had biting insects (or other families of bugs) as carriers. From the fleas carrying black plague throughout Europe to the malaria carrying mosquito that took the life of Alexander the Great, insect bites should not be taken lightly. Many unexplained itches and tiny sores on sleepers have been due to nocturnal flying and crawling bugs attracted by body heat and body gases. These insects can remain dormant in an unattended dwelling for years awaiting their next (or first) meal. They often produce anesthetic in their saliva which prevents detection while they chew through the skin to reach blood rich tissues. Feeding on the blood of the host, these creatures cross contaminate healthy individuals with infected animals they have just left. As human populations are increasing, more blood born diseases are being identified all the time. All efforts to control and repel the carriers should be taken. See the section on Air Purification in this book. For more information, call *HEALTH TALK* and consult topics 18, 19 and 88.

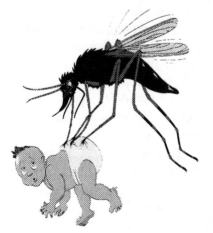

TREATMENT: When staying in a cabin or beach house, immediately fumigate the area with 10 drops of *T36-C7* in a pan of boiling water. The insect repellant properties of

Melaleuca oil are international. Apply *T36-C7* to children's clothing when going to natural parks or walking in the forest in the Spring. Inspect your children and yourself daily for small breaks in the skin indicating bites. Apply *T36-C7, Mela-Gel* or *Triple Antibiotic Ointment* and cover with a band aid for 24 hours.

INSOMNIA

Insomnia is a condition characterized by the inability of a person to fall asleep or wakefulness in the middle of the night. Some of the possible causes are a stressful lifestyle, indigestion, over-excitement, pain, discomfort, coffee or other stimulants, or drugs. Insomnia may also result from psychological origins such as mental illnesses, fears, or depression. Nutrition plays a big part. Neurohormones produced in the brain regulate the quantity and quality of our sleep. The elderly, as a group, are more prone to insomnia than younger people because of night-time bathroom calls. See the section on Fatigue in this book. For more information, call *HEALTH TALK* and consult topics 1, 66 and 69.

TREATMENT: General good health is the best approach in preventing insomnia. Sleeping pills cause unconsciousness but seldom bring restful sleep without side effects. *"Sleep is the reward for living a good day."* Avoid caffeine, nicotine, alcohol, sugar and a sedentary lifestyle. Regular daily exercise, deep breathing, drinking most liquids early in the day and practicing a philosophy that lives life in one-day segments are good habits to insure good sleep. A relaxing walk after dinner helps digestion and promotes good sleep. A glass of warm milk immediately before bed may be helpful. Milk contains an active amino acid (tryptophan) that causes the release of a brain hormone (serotonin) that allows sleep. Taking *The Vitality Pak* and Cell Wise with each meal and *Sustain Drink* while being active, will prevent the body from becoming imbalanced in neurohormone production.

ITCHING AND FLAKING SKIN

Itching and flaking skin can be caused by several different health concerns. Those suffering from psoriasis or allergies can experience itchy and flaky skin. This condition may also be seen in people whose diet is deficient in essential oils and some who are post-menopausal. See the sections on Allergic Reactions and Psoriasis in this book. For more information, call *HEALTH TALK* and consult topics 19, 20, 88 and 95.

TREATMENT: Bathe with *Natural Spa & Bath Oil*. Wash with *Gold Bar*. Apply *Body Satin Lotion* or *Problem Skin Lotion* to troubled areas. See your natural physician for further instructions.

JOCK ITCH

Fungal infections of the groin, commonly known as Jock Itch, can form ring lesions around the sides of the crotch. Scratching of the area can cause secondary infections or chronic dermatitis. The lesions may be complicated by a secondary bacteria or yeast such as candida. The occurrences are chronic since the fungus may persist indefinitely or may repeatedly infect susceptible individuals. It occurs more often during the summer or when humidity is high.

TREATMENT: Bathing in 1 oz of *Sol-U-Mel* and using the Antibiotic Liquid Soap or *Gold Bar* is helpful in controlling the fungus. After pat drying, apply *T36-C7* and *Mela-Gel* or *Triple Antibiotic Ointment*. *Problem Skin Lotion* may be used at bedtime. If irritation occurs, or if there is no improvement, discontinue and consult your natural physician.

KIDNEY STONES

Kidney stones can be formed in the kidneys, ureter, bladder, prostate or urethra. Their movement down the urinary tract can produce pain, bleeding, obstruction, and secondary infection. Milk drinkers and those who do not drink enough water tend to make stones from super-saturated urine. Patients who have passed stones describe them as *"a red hot bowling ball with razor blades"* while others say it is *"ten times worse than having a baby."* One third of a million Americans are hospitalized each year with kidney stones. Some people have had 3 or more surgeries over the years for stones. Modern ultrasound shattering (lithotripsy) is being performed but can damage the kidneys, spleen and lymph nodes as well. Since their formation conforms to the rules of chemistry, they can usually be prevented. About 80% of stones in Americans are composed of calcium salts, about 5% are uric acid, and 2% are made up of the amino acid cystine, with the rest made up of a mixture of phosphates released during infections or from medications. Many stones are *"silent"* until they begin to move. Some produce back pain or radiating pains into the groin area. Occasionally there is nausea, chills, fever and abdominal swelling.

TREATMENT: **If there is a family or personal history of stone formation, avoid dairy products completely. Drink plenty of water and 2 to 6 cups of *G'Day Melaleuca Tea* per day. Take *The Vitality Pak* with each meal. Ask your druggist about the side effects of all medications you are prescribed. If back or abdominal pain is present, apply *Pain-A-Trate* to the affected area along with a hot pad. Take a long hot bath. The stone passes easier if you are relaxed and comfortable.**

LEG CRAMPS

Leg cramps are due to either a deficiency in circulating calcium or reduced oxygen to muscles. Muscle cramps tend to appear after unconditioned physical activity. An irritated muscle can only do one thing- contract, which causes the cramp.

TREATMENT: **Stretching a *"crampy"* muscle can prevent knotting. Exercise in three steps - warm up for 5 minutes to stretch muscles - do your work out - then, cool down by moving slower or walking until the heart returns to your pre-exercise rate. Take *The Vitality Pak* with each meal. Drink *G'Day Melaleuca Tea* and *Sustain Drink* before, during and after exercise to reduce stress on the body.**

Take Cell Wise with each meal to properly oxygenate muscle cells during exercise without free radical formation. Persons who are bed ridden may need the assistance of external pneumatic compression boots to maximize circulation and prevent leg pains. Consult your natural physician.

LEUKOPLAKIA

Leukoplakia are white lesions on the skin inside the mouth. They are occasionally precancerous. While no certain cause is known, suspicion is aimed toward chemical irritations from smoking tobacco, chewing tobacco, food additives, food preservatives, food colorings, and dental materials, as well as toothpastes, mouthwashes and oral medications that contain alcohol which tend to dry the mucosa. When I started in practice, only a few elderly persons presented this condition. Lately, the number of teens and young adults with this is getting alarming.

TREATMENT: Get examined by your natural physician. Discontinue contact of questionable substances to the oral mucosa. Use *Tooth Polish* and *Breath-Away* or *Hot Shot Mouth & Throat Spray*. Drink 2 to 6 cups of *G'Day Melaleuca Tea* daily. Take *The Vitality Pak* with each meal.

LIVER DISORDERS

The liver is the master chemist of the body. Every bite of food, every ounce of non-food chemicals (Americans ingest about 11 pounds per year), and every waste product of the cells in the body is processed through the liver. The liver is so vital to life that we have been given one that is seven times larger than needed. Yes, we could actually have six-sevenths removed surgically and still live. The liver would respond by growing to its original size - a feat that no other organ can do. Besides genetic defects, disorders of the liver are classified into two main types - toxic and infectious. Liver toxicity occurs from alcohol consumption as well as storing substances in the liver that are unable to be detoxified. Infectious damage occurs from such conditions as mononucleosis, hepatitis and parasites. Once the liver is damaged, it begins to affect every other function and system of the body. Protecting the liver is a vital concern in these days of environmental pollution and untreatable infectious diseases.

PREVENTION: Drink plenty of purified water. Prepare food in a safe manner and demand safe handling by food establishments. Drink 2 to 4 cups of *G'Day Melaleuca Tea* each day. Take *The Vitality Pak* with each meal. NOTE: Allowing the liver to detoxify is essential for health. You cannot believe the reports patients have given after detoxifying their liver. Our great grand mothers used to give the family sulfur and molasses, along with cod liver oil, each spring. Unless you are a child, pregnant, nursing or hypoglycemic, you may want to do a Spring and Fall liver cleanse. Eat only raw, steamed, or juiced vegetables or vegetable soup and rice for one week. Drink one quart of apple juice along with 2 to 6 cups of *G'Day Melaleuca Tea* each day. On the sixth and seventh day, take one fourth to one half cup of olive oil followed by 1 tablespoon of Epsom salt dissolved in citrus juice. Stay close to home those days. Some nausea may occur due to the release of bile. Contact your natural physician if you have questions.

LONGEVITY

The human body and mind are designed to last one hundred and twenty years. Illnesses, stress, and accidents can shorten that span. Much of our ability to live a full and active life has to do with planning to be well and taking disease preventive measures early in life. The *Vitality For Life Personal Health Risk Appraisal* is an excellent place to start and should be performed and followed by everyone. What you do with this information, to a great extent, will determine the quality and quantity of your life through minimizing risks and maximizing wellness.

LYME DISEASE

As man invades forests for living space and also wishes to keep things *"natural,"* a new ecological balance between man and the environment takes place. Left to themselves, deer, mice and ticks have gotten along nicely with a parasitic organism called *Borrelia burgdorferi* for a long time. In 1975, a strange illness appeared with symptoms of inflammation and lesions on the skin, followed weeks later with nerve, heart and joint destruction. Many cases showed up in a rural community near Lyme, Connecticut. Researchers found that the newly discovered parasite needed the mouse and tick to grow on and required the deer for the adult to thrive. Removing any one of these three would stop the spread of the disease. Forty three states, areas of Europe, China, Japan, and Australia have the disease. The disease in humans starts with a tick bite causing a red macule or papule (usually on the thigh, buttock or under the arm) that grows over a few weeks up to 10 inches across then slowly disappears leaving the chronic symptoms. See the section on Insect Bites in this book.

TREATMENT: **Prevention is the best way to deal with this condition. If a tick bite is suspected, apply *T36-C7* every 4 hours until irritation subsides. *Triple Antibiotic Ointment* and *Mela-Gel* should be applied morning and evening under a band aid. For further assistance, contact your natural physician.**

MACULAR DEGENERATION

Macular degeneration is the deterioration of the central focal region of the back of the eye called the macula, resulting in impaired vision. The symptoms can be gradual or sudden, with objects usually appearing distorted in one eye. Upon examination, degeneration is often found in the normal appearing eye as well. Both men and women, mostly elderly, contract this condition and seldom have any other eye problems. There may be a hereditary link. Since the condition involves lack of nurturing of this normally blood-rich tissue, some scientists believe it is similar to brain tissue degeneration taking place in senility and atherosclerosis. See the sections on Atherosclerosis and Cardiovascular Disease in this book. Laser treatments are often used to treat advanced cases.

TREATMENT: **Have a *Vitality For Life Personal Health Risk Appraisal* performed and begin following the lifestyle advice. Take *The Vitality Pak* with each meal. Take *ProVex*** or *ProVex-Plus* daily to promote vascular integrity. Drink 2 to 4 cups of *G'Day Melaleuca Tea* each day. If you are older than 60, get a visual field evaluation test performed by your eye doctor every year.

MASSAGE

One of the oldest and most widely practiced health preserving therapies known is massage (See Bathing). Part of its benefits are the mechanical affect of *"rubbing"* and *"kneading"* tensions from the body. Many times we are unaware of these tensions until we are actually being massaged. Often, we can massage certain muscles on our own bodies. But, I feel that the greatest benefit is when it is done by a trained pair of gentle hands. There are several different techniques, each having certain advantages in specific situations. I recommend massage, especially for those who are bedridden or who are unable to exercise. Well muscled people can usually withstand more vigorous techniques, while those with less muscle will be comfortable with more gentle techniques. Modern massage therapists are trained in multiple techniques to meet your level of need and comfort.

TREATMENT: Start by taking a hot bath with 1 to 2 oz of *Natural Spa & Bath Oil* for 20 to 30 minutes. Feel the smoothness to your skin. The person receiving the massage must be in a comfortable position, usually face down. The person giving the massage must not feel hurried or uncomfortable when bending at the waist. Use ample amounts of warmed *Body Satin Lotion* to one extremity, neck, upper back, or lower back area at a time. Rub *Pain-A-Trate* into tender muscles and over stiff or painful joints. A few drops of *T36-C7* can be massaged into areas that feel cold and need better circulation. Massage the limbs toward the heart area, not away from the center of the body. When done gently, you can do no harm.

MEASLES

Rubeola, also known as seven-day measles is a highly contagious viral infection characterized by fever, bronchial cough, sneezing and irritated eyes that are sensitive to light. White spots inside the cheeks next to the first or second molars, known as Koplik's spots, appear 1 or 2 days before the rash begins. The brownish-red rash starts around the ears, on the face and neck, then spreads over the trunk and occasionally the limbs and usually lasts 4 to 7 days. Incubation is 7 to 14 days. It is easily transmitted from 2 to 4 days before the rash, and from 2 to 5 days after the rash disappears. In most cases, a person only has the measles once. Some people who are weakened by the measles suffer complications such as lung or middle ear infections. See the section on Rubella in this book.

TREATMENT: In well nourished children and adults, measles usually passes without complications. In malnourished or unhealthy individuals, great care must be taken to prevent a weakened immune system. Preventing ear infections (see the section on Earaches in this book), bacterial infections, and pneumonia is a primary goal. To prevent respiratory complications, use a warm steam vaporizer in the person's room using _T36-C7_ with them. Drink _G'Day Melaleuca Tea_ 3 to 6 times each day.

MENOPAUSE

The change of life for a woman should be celebrated with her husband one year after her last menses. This marks the end of child bearing and the beginning of mentoring of younger women. Menopause (stopping of flow) may be natural (average age 45 to 51), artificial (radiation or surgical) or premature (illness or stress induced). In a state of health, natural menopause has mild symptoms as the ovaries cease producing eggs and shrivel up like gray colored prunes. When a woman undergoes premature menopause, there are underlying causes which need specific attention. The greatest concern during and for about 5 years after menopause is the rapidly dwindling levels of estrogen to the cells of the body. Various lifestyle factors can have a great effect on estrogen production at this time of life, including stress vs. rest cycles.

Hot Flashes (See Hot Flashes), sweating, or light headedness affects about 75% of menopausal women and lasts for about 1 year. About 25 to 50% of these women have these symptoms for about 5 years or more. Other symptoms of tiredness, weight gain, headaches, irritability, insomnia and nervousness may be related to both estrogen deprivation and the stress of aging and changing lifestyle roles. Lack of sleep due to disturbances from hot flashes makes the fatigue and irritability worse. Occasional dizziness, numb or tingling sensations, palpitations and fast heart rate may occur. The risk of heart disease increases. Urinary incontinence, and urinary tract infections increase. Nausea, low bowel gas, constipation or diarrhea, joint and muscle pains are also common complaints. The major health risk is osteoporosis (See Osteoporosis) at this time. Preventing this problem should be every woman's primary health concern now. For more information, call *HEALTH TALK* and consult topic 75.

TREATMENT: Have a *Vitality For Life Personal Health Risk Appraisal* performed and begin following the advice for controlling stress. Take *The Vitality Pak* with each meal. Begin a daily exercise program using the *Access Bar* and *Sustain Drink* to prevent low blood sugar and fatigue. Drink 2 to 4 cups of *G'Day Melaleuca Tea* each day to prevent urinary tract infections. Communication is very important during this time. Overwork and continued stress can prolong symptoms.

MONONUCLEOSIS

The presence of fatigue, fever, sore throat and enlarged lymph nodes signifies the illness known as *"Mono"* which is caused by the Epstein-Barr virus. About 50% of children contact the virus before the age of five and have mild or no symptoms. Recovery is rapid. When infection occurs in young adults, an immune system battle results, where damage is done to human lymphocytes, spleen and the liver. Relapses are common if activity is resumed too soon. Many high school and college students miss school, because of not heeding the necessary *"rest-and-recover"* treatment. No medicines are known to treat this illness.

The incubation time of the virus is not fully known, but one week to two months is common. The illness can take up to three months to run its course. Complications can occur if it is not properly treated. *"Mono"* can go on to cause seizures, meningitis, psychosis, chronic fatigue syndrome, respiratory disease, jaundice, and hepatitis. Blood testing can detect past infections for several years after the illness has passed. For more information, call *HEALTH TALK* and consult topics 18 and 33. You may wish to see my educational video tape on Viral Infections.

TREATMENT: Complete bed rest for the first several weeks is often necessary to ease symptoms and prevent complications. Mild activity with mid-day rest periods is recommended for the first 4 to 6 weeks. Drink 2 to 6 cups of *G'Day Melaleuca* tea each day. Take the *Vitality Pak* with juice or broth for the first 2 to 3 weeks, then with meals. Breathe *T36-C7* enriched steam vapor to prevent respiratory complications. Hot baths with 1 oz of *Sol-U-Mel* and 1 oz of *Natural Spa & Bath Oil* for 30 minutes are helpful in the absence of a fever. Do not do heavy lifting, bending at the waist or jumping for 3 months as permanent damage to the liver or spleen may occur.

MORNING SICKNESS

On about the tenth day after conception, the developing placenta begins producing the hormones HCG and estrogen, which may cause mild to severe nausea and vomiting in susceptible mothers-to-be. It can last up to the 4th month. This, along with tender breasts and no menstrual period, are strong (but not absolute) evidence of pregnancy. A self administered pregnancy test can be performed on urine, and they are now sensitive enough to be accurate only a few days after conception. For more information, call *HEALTH TALK* and consult topic 39.

TREATMENT: There are no FDA approved drugs for morning sickness. Any anti-nausea drugs can cause damage to the developing baby. Drink and eat small amounts of bland

foods (steamed vegetables, baked potato, dry bread, etc.) throughout the day to not stretch the stomach and trigger the very sensitive gag reflex. The first food and drink should be before getting out of bed in the morning. *Sustain Drink* is a helpful supplement at this time. Small amounts of *G'Day Melaleuca Tea* taken throughout the day are very calming to the stomach. The need for vitamin B6 and magnesium is great and can be supplied from *The Vitality Pak* (they may need to be ground up and put in a drink). Ginger is a very good herb for controlling nausea and has no side effects. The use of wrist straps fitted with acupressure beads help some women with morning sickness.

MUCOUS

Thin, watery mucous is a product of healthy membranes in the body and is needed to protect soft tissues from damaging environmental substances. Sudden cold air can cause the normal release of excess mucous from the nasal sinuses. Thick, discolored or stringy sputum (phlegm), vaginal, eye, stool or nasal mucous is a sign of irritation or infection. Mild bacterial growth, viruses, chronic yeast or fungal infections, digestive problems, stress, allergies and chemical sensitivities can produce this type of mucous.

TREATMENT: Drink 2 to 6 cups of *G'Day Melaleuca Tea* each day to reduce the number of harmful organisms in the bowel and urinary tract. Breathe steam inhalation with *T36-C7* to clear tear ducts, nasal and sinus mucous membranes. Douche with *Nature's Cleanse* as directed to reduce vaginal viruses, yeast, molds, fungus and bacteria. Repeat any of the above to maintain healthy mucous.

NAUSEA

The unpleasant feeling that one is about to vomit is part of a regulatory mechanism that allows for expulsion of potentially harmful substances. Nausea is often associated with improper body functions including constipation or gall bladder congestion. It can also be due to such conditions as pregnancy, the flu, bad food, some drugs, confusion of the balance mechanism of the middle ear by irregular motion, a ruptured inner ear membrane, or spinal nerve irritation from vertebral misalignment. Vomiting is the forceful expulsion of the stomach contents produced from involuntary contraction of abdominal muscles. Psychological factors such as *"distasteful"* food can cause nausea with vomiting. Physical stress such as running too fast, children throwing temper tantrums, or strong coughing can induce vomiting. For more information, call *HEALTH TALK* and consult topics 39, 40 and 86. See the sections on Constipation and Indigestion in this book.

TREATMENT: Determine the cause. People can get nauseated after taking their supplements either at or between meals. Food in the stomach helps to mix the contents of the tablets so they do not concentrate nutrients on the nerve sensitive mucosal lining of the stomach. Contact your natural physician if medical advise is needed.

NERVOUSNESS

"A sound mind in a sound body" was the Greek ideal for a healthy person. We now know that what impairs one part of our being will affect the other. Nervousness (mild anxiety) can be due to worry about an unfounded or unlikely situation or event. Deprivation of sleep, clinical depression, and the aches and pains that often accompany tense muscles are typical with nervous people. Nervousness tends to be a learned behavior that depletes the body of valuable nutrients, which in turn perpetuate the condition. Chemical addictions, including nicotine (nervous stimulant) and alcohol (nervous depressant), as well as long term prescription drugs, should be avoided and corrected before permanent improvement can take place. A healthy body makes its own chemicals for awareness and response to real problems. It is one way the body responds to stress. Nearly all mental disorders include nervousness as a component of the diagnosis. For more information, call *HEALTH TALK* and consult topics 63-70. See the section on Exercise in this book.

TREATMENT: Have a *Vitality For Life Personal Health Risk Appraisal* performed and follow the results for stress

control, exercise, and diet. Take *The Vitality Pak* with each meal. Drink 2 to 4 cups of *G'Day Melaleuca Tea* each day. Practice relaxation and breathing exercises each day. Believe that you can train your body, with help, to be less nervous.

NICOTINE WITHDRAWAL

We are often asked, *"How can I quit smoking?"* The answer is different for each individual. Some people make up their mind to quit and have no symptoms of withdrawal. Others have neurological and psychological symptoms typical of drug addiction. Depression, anxiety, and behavioral changes are common. Since nicotine is of the alkaloid family, along with morphine and codeine, chemical detoxification and needed emotional support are important to recovery. The appetite suppressive effects of nicotine are well known. Compulsive eating during recovery must be compensated for with exercise and adequate nutrition.

TREATMENT: Have a *Vitality For Life Personal Health Risk Appraisal* performed and begin following the advice. Take *The Vitality Pak* with each meal and drink 2 to 4 cups of *G'Day Melaleuca Tea* each day. Eat one *This Is Fiber?* bar each day to speed detoxification. Exercise and drink plenty of water. If needed, do not hesitate to get professional guidance. If congestion exists, use *CounterAct*, 1 tablet 3-4 times per day.

NUTRITION

Nutrition is more than just getting enough food. It is getting enough of the right food at the right time for the prevailing needs of the body. It is the miracle the body performs when changing the molecular structure of food into living human tissue. Everyone has slightly different needs for nutrition based upon genetics, lifestyle, temperament, geographic location, past illnesses, digestive and absorptive capacity, and stress effects. The best thing you can do (after choosing the right parents) is to determine your unique nutritional needs. Waiting until you have a health problem before getting concerned about nutrition is like waiting until your car engine runs out of oil to become interested in engine lubrication. Just Do It!

Not getting enough food is called malnutrition. On the average, Americans are over fed and under nourished. I use the term dysnutrition in this condition. Choosing *"brands"* that are heavily advertised in place of foods in their original state is due to clever marketing and advertising techniques. An example is potato chips in place of eating a baked potato.

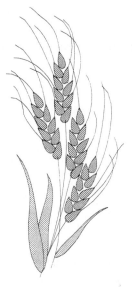

Why is the topic of nutrition so important to us? The Surgeon General's Report in 1990 disclosed that "...*eighty percent of all current diseases are due to chronic degenerative states in the body either directly or indirectly related to diet and nutrition.*" Twenty five years ago, in spite of volumes of published clinical studies, medical scientists lacked *"conclusive"* evidence that cancer and heart disease (number 1 and 2 leading causes of death) were related to diet. More recently, only a few physicians would deny that diet and nutrition are the leading cause and the best prevention for these conditions. My chiropractic training awakened me to the powerful advantage better nutrition gives. This sudden awakening of the public to the *"new"* nutrition has paved the way for fad diets, quick vitamin cures and over night experts who have had little training and often less experience in using nutrition as *"the"* first medicine of choice. As Hippocrates said, *"Let your medicine be your food and let your food be your medicine."* This should not be too difficult to understand.

PRACTICE: The *Vitality For Life Personal Health Risk Appraisal* is a good place to start. **Learn where your weaknesses are and design a plan to prevent illness. Take** *The Vitality Pak* **with each meal. Drink** *G'Day Melaleuca Tea* **daily. Get enough rest. Learn how to relax. Practice playful activities (those that make you talk, laugh and breathe deeply) every day. The desire for self nurturing exists when body, mind and spirit are healthy. Some people may need a little help to get started.**

OBESITY

The underlying causes of clinical obesity (being more than 20 per cent above your optimum weight, or having more than 40 per cent of your body weight as fat) often stems from boredom eating, stressful eating, childhood or sexual abuse, drug effects or dysnutrition. See the section on Nutrition in this book. Less than 10% of the cases of obesity I see involve glandular conditions. The obvious problem is in storing more calories than are being burned through metabolic needs and exercise. All chronic degenerative diseases are accelerated when obesity is present.

Our ancestors earned and burned about 4,000 to 6,000 calories each day just in living, working and walking to school. Because of our automated life style, we earn and burn between 1,200 and 2,000 calories each day. Our nutrient needs for vitamins, minerals and cofactors common to food remain the same. What is wrong with this picture?

I see people every week who have lost hundreds of pounds over the years only to gain it right back. This is due to a physiological condition called *"set point."* The hypothalamus gland in the brain constantly monitors the temperature of the inside of the body compared with the outside surface of the body. The appetite center, also located in the hypothalamus, is activated when factors begin to lower blood sugar. Our bodies are then conditioned or *"set"* to burn less when apparent reserves begin to drop. We actually slow down our rate of calorie burning to conserve fuel. This is why people can go on a water diet for a week and not loose more than one or two pounds. Fatigue is the most common complaint when total calories are restricted. What must happen is to change the set point so that the body is satisfied with less intake while it is burning more of its reserves. The nutrient Adenosine is a key to releasing fat stores while satisfying the body's nutrient needs. Body fat is deficient in this nutrient. Adding dietary adenosine selectively speeds fat burning. Restricting dietary fats to less than 20% of daily intake decreases free radicals and hunger sensations. Exercise speeds up the process of weight loss by burning the least needed tissue first - fat. Continuing exercise establishes a new set point which is the permanent way to control weight. See the section on Exercise in this book. For more information, call *HEALTH TALK* and consult topic 3.

TREATMENT: Have a *Vitality For Life Personal Health Risk Appraisal* performed and begin following the advice. Eat an *Access Bar* 15 minutes before exercise. Plan your meals ahead of time. Remove all unhealthy snack foods from your home. Use exercise as a means of handling stress instead of eating. If childhood stresses are present to *"any"* extent, contact Over Eaters Anonymous and get involved. This non-profit group is an excellent source of free support. If necessary, see a counselor or a natural physician for appetite suppressive herbs, acupuncture, or specific metabolic testing. Seeking help in getting started is far better than reading a HOW TO book and doing it alone. They don't work for 99% of people who buy them. The weight simply slips back, with interest!

OSGOOD-SCHLATTER'S DISEASE

Young athletes have muscles that are stronger than the actual bone to which they are attached. Heavy track and field events, especially broad jumping, put unusual strain on the thigh muscles as they connect with the tibia just below the knee. Some young athletes develop this crippling disorder due to an avulsion (fracture) which tears away soft bone with pain and swelling of the area. Once called *"growing pains"*, knee supports were used to prevent injuries to 14 thru 18 year olds.

TREATMENT: Apply an ice pack for 5 to 10 minutes to acute pain areas. Take *MELA-CAL* with each meal, before and after exercise to maximize bone development. Take *MEL-VITA* with each meal to enhance growth and healing of injuries. Apply *Pain-A-Trate* directly to the affected area before and after exercise to minimize swelling and pain. Rub exercised thigh muscles with *Pain-A-Trate* to relax tension and stimulate circulation. Jacuzzi or whirlpool massage is excellent for reducing tension. Do not over-train. You have a long life ahead of you.

OSTEOARTHRITIS

A degeneration of joint material including cartilage and bone takes place when complex systems of mechanical injury, biological stress, biochemical irritation, and enzymatic or nutritional deficiencies are upset. There is no single cause for osteoarthritis. Healthy joints have such little friction that without some precipitating condition, they will never wear out. Apparently the amount of friction in the joint increases after repetitive injury (plucking chickens), taking drugs for other conditions (many drugs affect joint and bone metabolism), toxic reactions to environmental pollution (pesticides, herbicides, food additives, etc.), trace nutrient deficiencies, or dietary habits that promote nutritional deficiencies (excessive coffee drinking, alcohol, limited diet selection, etc.). Osteoarthritic joints have less flexible cartilage and more infiltrated bone causing the tell-tail enlarged joints on fingers. Exercise tends to pump nutrients in and wastes out of healthy cartilage. See the section on Arthritis in this book.

TREATMENT: Exercise and movement is imperative. A number of my patients who complained of painful hands, especially in cold weather, found relief by taking up knitting. Start each morning by doing the evening snack dishes by hand in hot water. Apply *Pain-A-Trate* to the affected joints. Take *The Vitality Pak* with each meal. Take *ProVex* or *ProVex-Plus* daily for cartilage growth. Drink 2 to 4 cups of *G'Day Melaleuca Tea* each day. Consult your natural physician.

OSTEOPOROSIS

There are two major types of osteoporosis, primary and secondary. The primary type occurs more often in women and progresses with age. Known as the *"shrinking disease"*, it affects more women over the age of 65 than breast and uterine cancer combined. The loss of calcium prematurely is due to a combination of factors. Women who are of slight build, smoke cigarettes, consume caffeine, fail to exercise, and do not ingest enough calcium are prone to develop fractures of large weight bearing bones after menopause. The spine, pelvis, and femoral hip joint areas are most often affected. School aged girls are deficient in dietary calcium. Studies show that only 58% of teen age girls consume the recommended daily allowance of calcium. The rest are at great risk of never attaining 100% of their expected bone calcium density. Since the expected life span of a woman born in the 1990's is 90 + years, more emphasis should be placed on teaching girls how to prevent this disease.

Secondary osteoporosis is less common and can be due to malabsorption of calcium, endocrine imbalances, prescription or other drug reactions, liver disease, or kidney disease. If you are having any of these problems, consult your natural physician for specific advice.

TREATMENT: Have a *Vitality For Life Personal Health Risk Appraisal* performed and begin following the advice. If you are a woman of menopausal age and have lost 1/2 inch or more height since you were 18, begin a program to minimize osteoporosis. If more than 1 inch of height has been lost, consult your natural physician for a calcium metabolism evaluation. Take *The Vitality Pak* with each meal to insure adequate trace nutrients. Drink 2 to 4 cups of *G'Day Melaleuca Tea* each day to detoxify. Take *ProVex* or *ProVex-Plus* daily. The ingredients in the *ProVex* products are powerful stabilizers of collagen structures, which is the major protein structure in bone.

Paronychia

Paronychia is an infection of the tissues around a fingernail or toenail. It is caused by yeast such as *Candida albicans* or bacteria such as *Pseudomonas* or *Proteus*. It enters through a break in the skin. The infection may follow the nail margin and may extend beneath the nail where the infection penetrates more deeply into the finger or toe. Tissue breakdown into the tendons and muscle in the finger or toe may result. Eventually the infected nail may become distorted and loose normal function if not treated promptly.

TREATMENT: Early detection and treatment is important. Wash the affected area with *Antibacterial Liquid Soap* and soak for 15 minutes in 1 quart of warm water and 1 oz of *Sol-U-Mel*. Pat dry. Apply *T36-C7* to the fingernail or toenail morning and night then follow with *Triple Antibiotic Ointment* or *Mela-Gel*. Cover the area with a loose bandage. Chronic infections may require repeated applications for several months. If *Candida albicans* is the causative agent in a female, douching with *Nature's Cleanse* may be needed to reduce the fungus. Drink *G'Day Melaleuca Tea* 2 to 4 times each day.

Poison Ivy, Poison Oak, Poison Sumac

Complex chemical agents in certain plants are capable of producing acute dermatitis in sensitized individuals. Poison ivy, poison oak or sumac's blistery rash is a result of coming in contact with the plant itself, or handling the clothing of someone who has been in contact with it. Some people are more sensitive to the oily plant juices than others. Many substances other than poison oak, poison ivy or sumac cause this acute reaction, including ragweed and primrose. Shoe dyes, formaldehyde in clothing, penicillin, sulfonamides, neomycin, anesthetics, food stabilizers and cosmetics can also produce severe dermatitis.

TREATMENT: Immediate removal of the affecting agent is necessary for any treatment to be effective. Immediately wash the area thoroughly with *Antibacterial Liquid Soap* and warm water. Pat (don't rub) dry. Apply *Triple Antibiotic Ointment* and cover with a loose gauze bandage three times each day until resolved. If the rash or blistering has appeared before treatment can be started, soak gauze bandages in cool *G'Day Melaleuca Tea* and cover the affected area. Re-soak gauze and apply every 15 minutes until pain subsides. Apply *Triple Antibiotic Ointment* three times each day until resolved. Draining the blisters can be done but do not remove the covering skin. If pain does not reduce, apply *Pain-A-Trate*. Contact your natural physician if improvement is not seen after 4 days.

POLYPS

This is a clinical term which refers to any mass of tissue that protrudes from a mucous membrane in the nose, throat, vocal chord, ear, bowel, vagina, or urinary tract tissue and extends outward. It may be normal tissue or diseased. While there is no known cause of polyps, reactions to certain drugs, pollutants or irritants seems linked. I have had allergy patients who had used nasal inhalers for years to reduce congestion and demonstrated polyps in their nose. Most cancers of the bowel start from a polyp. (Rectal screening by your natural physician should be performed as part of your annual physical examination if you are over 50 years old)

TREATMENT: Bleeding polyps should be seen by your natural physician. Only easily accessed polyps can be treated at home. Apply *Mela-Gel* or *Problem Skin Lotion* three times each day for 14 days to polyps. If reduction does not occur, see your natural physician.

PREGNANCY

Pregnancy is a natural process, yet one out of every eleven pregnancies produces an abnormal baby. The best thing to do to have a healthy happy baby is to have healthy happy parents. External factors that are known to greatly affect a normal pregnancy include the nutrition of the mother and the safety of the environment. Exercise should be continued during pregnancy to maintain muscle tone and prevent back problems from the added 20 to 30 pounds of normal weight gain.

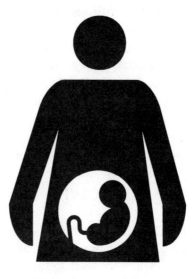

Since the baby is made from molecular building blocks, maximizing nutritional needs and minimizing non-nutritional chemicals is vital. Nutritional needs of the expectant mother increase for all of the known nutrients. A lack of folic acid is now known to cause spinal cord defects in babies of deficient mothers. It is estimated that 85% to 90% of all pregnant women take prescription or over-the-counter drugs during their pregnancy, with 3% to 12% of abnormal pregnancies resulting from their side effects. Drugs and babies do not mix well. Neither does carbon monoxide from cigarette smoke, alcohol, or fumes from paint or toxic house-hold cleaners. Actually, common sense gives us good direction in avoiding these things. The heightened sense of smell and taste during pregnancy gives a woman a great defense for her baby. See the sections on Nausea or Morning Sickness in this book.

TREATMENT: Plan for your baby at least one year before you intend to get pregnant. Have a *Vitality For Life Personal Health Risk Appraisal* performed and follow the advice. Exercise for 30 minutes daily - walking is the best prior to the birth of the baby. *The Vitality Pak,* when taken three times a day, satisfies all of the minimum recommendations for 18 vitamins and minerals, including folate, during pregnancy. Eating low on the food pyramid automatically gives adequate roughage to prevent constipation and water retention. Toxemia during pregnancy is best prevented by minimizing stress while balancing activity with rest. See your natural physician for further advice.

PRURITIS ANI

Pruritis Ani is Latin for *"Itching Anus"*. This area of the body tends to have an almost built-in *"readiness to itch."* Itching around the anus can be caused from something as simple as pin worms in children, or as complicated as rectal cancer in adults. Internal hemorrhoids are often discovered as a cause in adults. Many causes stem from chemical irritation with perfumed soap or toilet tissue. Food allergies (particularly eggs or milk) are frequently associated with this condition and often produce a red ring around the anal opening. Food additive sensitivities (colorings, flavorings and preservatives) are among the most common in children. I have seen fungal growths such as *Candida albicans*, psychological responses in anxiety patients, other skin problems such as psoriasis or contact dermatitis, heavy coffee or cola drinking, poor hygiene and over meticulous cleaning with soaps and perfumed powder as causes of intense anal itching.

TREATMENT: Try to treat the cause. Soaking in a warm bath with 1 cup of Epsom salt and 1 oz of *Natural Spa & Bath Oil* often reduces anal muscle tightness, which contributes to the itch. Avoid applying or consuming chemical conditioned substances. Drink 2 to 6 cups of *G'Day Melaleuca Tea* each day. Take *The Vitality Pak* with each meal. *Pain-A-Trate* can be dabbed around the anus during extreme cases to minimize itching. *Problem Skin Lotion* often gives lasting relief from pruritus ani while the true cause is being corrected. If itching persists, consult your natural physician for further evaluation. If congestion exists, use *CounterAct*, 1 tablet 3-4 times per day.

PSORIASIS

Psoriasis is a chronic and recurrent disease of the skin which is characterized by dry, well circumscribed silvery scaling patches of various sizes. The patches can vary in severity from one or two lesions to a widespread dermatosis with disabling arthritis. The cause is unknown, but it appears to be related to inadequate detoxification possibly through the kidney or the alimentary tract. I have seen patients who developed psoriasis after prolonged use of over-the-counter pain medication which effected their kidneys. Thick scaling is probably due to an increased rate of epidermal cell growth. This cosmetic deformity proves socially embarrassing although it is not contagious.

Psoriasis usually involves the scalp and the upper surface of the extremities, particularly the elbows and knees, the back and the buttocks. The nails, eyebrows, armpits and abdomen or groin region may also be affected. Occasionally the illness is generalized. The lesions are more sharply localized and usually heal without scarring. Hair growth does not appear to be affected. Extension of lesions sometimes produces large plaques up to one-half of an inch thick. Nail involvement may resemble fungal infections, causing a separation of the nail with thickening and discoloration, and debris under the nail plate. Quite often, allergies, stress and environmental sensitivities should be evaluated. Nutritional needs tend to be elevated during this time.

TREATMENT: Bathe using *Antibacterial Liquid Soap* and soak in *Natural Spa & Bath Oil* for 30 minutes each night. Pat dry (don't rub). Apply *Problem Skin Lotion* to the scaly areas. Apply *T36-C7* to newly inflamed or red areas. Cover with *Mela-Gel*. Daily sunlight exposure for 15 to 20 minutes is helpful. Practice relaxation. Eat healthy food. Take *The Vitality Pak* with each meal and drink 2 to 6 cups of *G'Day Melaleuca Tea* daily. Consult your natural physician for further advice.

RASHES

Rashes can be caused by many things. They should be treated to prevent secondary infections and reduce any stinging or itching. See the section on Dermatitis in this book. For more information, call *HEALTH TALK* and consult topics 20 and 21.

TREATMENT: Take a hot bath with 1 oz of *Natural Spa & Bath Oil*, plus 1 oz of *Sol-U-Mel*, and soak for 20 to 30 minutes. Pat dry. Apply *Problem Skin Lotion, Triple Antibiotic Ointment,* or *Pain-A-Trate* to the affected area. One Air Force officer had suffered for 23 years with an extensive body rash he brought back from Viet Nam. He found that the *Problem Skin Lotion* gave him the most symptomatic relief during his slow recovery. He had been burned and poisoned from powerful prescription medications for years and had given up hope, scratching himself to sleep many a night in agony. He now praises these products to everyone he meets - rash free!

RINGWORM

A round, reddened, often bulls eye appearing rash anywhere on the skin is evidence of ringworm. This superficial infection is caused by dermatophytes fungus (those that invade only dead tissue of the skin, nails or hair). At least three different strains of fungi can cause ringworm. Household pets such as cats and dogs carry these fungi on their fur and skin. Some cases produce only mild inflammation and often go unnoticed and untreated, then gradually reappear in hot weather. Other types cause a sudden outbreak of a violent looking rash with vesicles and swelling of the tissue due to a strong immunological reaction of the body against the fungi. Severe itching, especially in the groin area (See Jock Itch) provokes scratching, which tends to spread the infection by the fingernails or causes skin damage and produces secondary infection from bacteria. Since differentiation of these types of fungi is difficult, these infections are approached according to the sites involved. Confirming a diagnosis is made by seeing your natural physician who will scrape a sample of the skin and either examine it under a microscope or send it to the lab for culture.

TREATMENT: As in most infections, prevention is the best thing to stop the spread of the infection. Family members must take precautions to not pick up the infection from another

family member. Always wear shower sandals when in public showers such as athletic locker rooms or in swimming pools where the fungi grow readily and cross with other strains. Bathe your cat and dog regularly with *Sol-U-Mel* during warm weather. Treat any pet rashes or *"hot spots"* with *T36-C7, Triple Antibiotic Ointment,* or *Mela-Gel.*

Apply *T36-C7, Mela-Gel* or *Triple Antibiotic Ointment* on any suspicious areas of the skin immediately after showering. Direct sunlight and thoroughly air drying the body after showering or swimming is a great preventive act also. Take *The Vitality Pak* with each meal to optimize trace nutrients. Drink 2 to 3 cups of *G'Day Melaleuca Tea* daily. Bathing is advised over showering. Always put 1 oz of *Sol-U-Mel,* along with *Natural Spa & Bath Oil* in the tub. Use a clean washcloth with the *Antibacterial Liquid Soap* or *Gold Bar.* Drink 2 to 6 cups of *G'Day Melaleuca Tea* daily. Apply *T36-C7* to any active or itching areas. Allow it to dry before applying *Mela-Gel* or *Triple Antibiotic Ointment.* Cracking or oozing skin should receive a generous amount of *Problem Skin Lotion.* Take *The Vitality Pak* of nutritional supplements regularly.

RUBELLA

(German Measles or Three-Day Measles) After 14 to 21 days from the time of exposure, susceptible persons will feel tired and may have slightly swollen lymph nodes under the eyes, behind the ears, and in the neck. Other symptoms include the development of a headache, moderate fever and runny nose and a fine textured pinkish rash which starts on the face and neck, moves to the trunk and limbs, and lasts about 3 days. The virus is spread through the air or by physical contact (See Air Purification). Rubella is much milder in children and adults than *"red"* measles, which not only differs in color of the rash from rubella but displays a painful cough and Koplik's spots on the inside of the mouth. (See Measles) Women in their first three months of pregnancy who are susceptible to rubella, can contract the virus (usually from children) and naturally abort or give birth to developmentally defective and often mentally retarded (congenital rubella) infants. In children up through teenagers, the illness is generally mild. Except for the risk of congenital rubella, some scientists question the risk/benefit ratio of immunizing children. Instead, some still see the wisdom of exposing 5 year olds to the useful institution of kindergarten where actually developing childhood diseases, in a well nourished environment, usually gives lifelong immunity. Immunizations offer no more than about 15 years of protection. Rubella may be difficult to properly determine without a trained physician using laboratory testing, as some of the symptoms can resemble other illnesses.

TREATMENT: Since the active virus can be spread from about one week before to one week after the eruption of the rash, epidemics of rubella sweep through susceptible children quickly. By then the virus has spread throughout the body. Only palliative care can be given to ease discomfort and prevent secondary infections such as pneumonia. Soaking in a hot bath with 1 ounce of *Natural Spa & Bath Oil* and 1 ounce *Sol-U-Mel* for 20 minutes may help diminish the rash. Chicken soup, *G'Day Melaleuca Tea* and *Vita-Bears* Children's Multiple Vitamin/Mineral Supplement is the ration of choice. More solid food can be given upon request which is usually after the rash subsides.

SAUNA BATH

The Scandinavians are right! I love the deep tissue cleansing that only sweating can give. Endurance exercises such as racket sports, aerobics, running and bicycling get the blood and perspiration flowing. Perspiration contains waste products dissolved in water that closely approximates urine in composition. Sauna temperatures of 170 to 200 degrees with moisture quickly open skin pores and speed the process of removing petro-chemicals, pesticides, herbicides and metabolic wastes which resist detoxification within the body. I recommend it to anyone who is not on heart medication, an uncontrolled diabetic, a small child or pregnant. See the section on Bathing in this book.

TREATMENT: Shower or bathe using Antibiotic Liquid Soap or *Gold Bar* to remove dirt and environmental chemicals from the skin and hair. Drink one quart of water or *G'Day*

Melaleuca Tea before entering a sauna. Drink one cup of cool water or *G'Day Melaleuca Tea* for every 5 minutes in the sauna to replace body fluid. Your weight after a sauna should be the same as before you started. First time sauna users or elderly persons should limit their use to only one span of 15 minutes, then shower normally. Veteran sauna bathers can take a cool shower (or jump in a snow bank) then return to the sauna for an additional 15 or 20 minutes for deep cleansing. NOTE: Never sauna alone! Immediately get out of sauna if dizziness, light headedness or shortness of breath are experienced. Contact your natural physician.

SENILITY (FAILING MEMORY)

Reduced blood flow and lessened oxygen tension within the frontal regions of the brain, as well as accumulation of heavy metals within the brain, are believed to cause premature senility in many people. While scientists have found a strong genetic link in the development of this problem, preventive measures should be taken early in life to postpone or avoid this loss of human creativity.

TREATMENT: Avoid toxic environments, old paint, aluminum products (aluminum cookware, deodorants containing aluminum, etc.), heavy fats and sugar. Ask your preventive minded doctor to perform a hair elemental analysis to find out if your health is threatened. Take *The Vitality Pak* and *Cell Wise Anti-Oxidants* with each meal. Drink 3 cups of *G'Day Melaleuca Tea* each day. Use *ProVex-Plus* to prevent and treat the early stages of this condition.

SCABIES

Scabies are transmittable parasitic infections characterized by intensive itching and secondary bacterial infections. They are caused by the itch mite known as *Sarcoptes scabiei* which burrows under the skin to feed and lay its eggs. The itching is usually noticed most intensely when the person is in bed. The characteristic initial lesions of the burrow are seen as fine wavy dark lines a few millimeters to a half inch long with a minute papule at the open end. A red lesion occurs on the finger webs, on the under-surface of the wrists, about the elbows and under arms, around the nipple area of the breasts in females, on the genitals in males, and along the belt line and on the lower buttocks. The face is not usually involved in adults, but may be in infants. The burrow may be difficult to find particularly when the disease is persistent for several weeks, because the burrow is often obscured by scratching or by secondary lesions. Diagnosis is confirmed by seeing the parasite under a microscope after a scraping is taken from the burrow. The mites can remain dormant in infected bed clothes or blankets for months awaiting a warm victim to bring them back to life. Scabies are nothing to ignore. See the section on Chiggers in this book. NOTE: Treatment of scabies with lindane containing medications (Kwell) have multiple hazards to children. Nervous system disturbances have been observed and reported in the scientific literature.

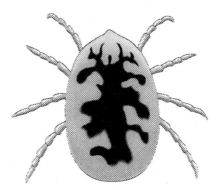

TREATMENT: Soak in a hot bath for 20 minutes each night with 1 oz of *Natural Spa & Bath Oil* and 1 oz of *Sol-U-Mel*. Apply *T36-C7* to the affected areas each morning and night. Apply *Problem Skin Lotion* or *Triple Antibiotic Ointment* to give long term protection against infection. Apply *Pain-A-Trate* to extremely itchy areas. If no improvement is observed within 7 days, contact your natural physician.

SCALDS

Hot water, steam, liquid nitrogen, or liquid propane can produce scalds. Immediate blistering and light colored skin is characteristic.

Care should be taken to not dislodge delicate superficial skin. Painful blisters may appear within a few minutes indicating second degree penetration. Loose, swollen skin without blistering is evidence of third degree penetration. See the section on Burns in this book.

TREATMENT: Immediately apply cold water to hot water scalds and warm water to cold scalds. Pat dry and apply *T36-C7* or *Pain-A-Trate* to the affected area. Wrap area with a sterile dressing. Begin treating as a second or third degree burn.

SCIATICA

Spinal misalignments in the low lumbar spine can cause mild to severe pain radiating along the sciatic nerve, which travels down the back of the leg, behind the knee, to the foot. Expert advice should be sought from your chiropractor, as sciatica may be a sign of degenerative disk disease. See the section on Back Pain in this book.

TREATMENT: Use a flexible elastic back brace when doing heavy lifting or prolonged bending. Get regular chiropractic check ups *before* a full blown attack develops. If low back muscle spasms or tension is present, usually after unusual activity, take 2 *MELA-CAL* every four hours until the pain is gone. Take *ProVex* or *ProVex-Plus* daily to relieve inflammation and promote healing. Apply ice for 5 to 10 minutes, followed by 15 to 20 minutes of heat every hour for the first 4 hours. Apply *Pain-A-Trate* to the affected area after each heat treatment. Avoid prolonged sitting. Try to lie down either on your back with a pillow under your knees or on your side with a pillow between your bent knees. To prevent sciatic pain, exercise the abdominal muscles by doing partial sit-ups (crunches) each morning and evening. This not only strengthens the lower abdominal muscle girdle but it helps maintain a good posture.

SEBORRHEA

This is a scaly inflammation of the skin which occurs around the scalp, face and occasionally other areas of the body. Seborrhea usually appears as dry or greasy scaling and is often mis-diagnosed as thick dandruff. In the most severe cases, a yellow or red scaling with papules around the rash appears usually along the hairline and behind the ears. It is often found in the ear canal, on the eyebrows, on the bridge of the nose, in the nasal folds, or on the upper chest. Seborrheic dermatitis does not cause hair loss. Infants in their first month of life may develop seborrheic dermatitis, often called cradle cap, which results in a thick yellow crusted scalp. In severe cases, cracks and yellow scaling behind the ears, and red facial papules may be present. Genetic and climatic factors, in addition to chemical and allergic sensitivities seem to affect the incidence and severity of the disease. The disease is more prevalent in the winter when more time is spent indoors and household chemicals are concentrated. I have seen some cases of seborrhea miraculously improve with the avoidance of coffee.

TREATMENT: Take *The Vitality Pak* with each meal. Drink 2 to 6 cups of *G'Day Melaleuca Tea* daily for detoxification. Bathe using *Antibacterial Liquid Soap* in a tub containing 1 oz of *Natural Spa & Bath Oil* and 1 oz of *Sol-U-Mel*. Shampoo with Melaleuca *Natural Shampoo* or *Herbal Shampoo* daily. Continue the bathing procedure once daily, but apply *T36-C7* with either *Problem Skin Lotion* or *Mela-Gel* after each bath.

SHINGLES

Shingles are caused by the same virus in adults that causes chickenpox in children. Shingles manifests as small, very painful clusters of blisters which form along a sensory nerve on the skin of the chest, neck, face, stomach or limbs. These pink or white blisters contain a clear fluid which may later become pus. They dry up and disappear in about a week, but the area feels irritated for longer.

TREATMENT: Shingles can be treated similarly to chickenpox, except for the use of more *Sol-U-Mel* and *Natural Spa & Bath Oil*, detoxification, and satisfying the increased nutritional need for B vitamins. Take *The Vitality Pak* with each meal. Drink 2 to 6 cups of *G'Day Melaleuca Tea* to reduce virus growth. Add 2 oz of Melaleuca *Natural Spa & Bath Oil* and 2 oz of *Sol-U-Mel* to a warm tub of water. Soak for 30 minutes. Pay dry. Apply a drop of *T36-C7* to pustules followed by *Triple Antibiotic Ointment*. Continue treatment once or twice daily for 6 days. Consult your natural physician if further advice is needed.

SINUS CONGESTION

Sinus congestion can be due to mild infections or generalized irritations caused from allergies, chronic airborne pollutants, cigarette smoking, dust, grasses, pollens or other chemicals. Often, bacterial sinus infections are caused by repeated use of antihistamines which dry mucous membranes and lead to severe susceptibility to other infections. Inflammation caused from mold sensitivity or anemia can also be the underlying cause. When frontal sinuses found above and behind the eyes are effected, headaches may occur. Coughing is often associated with deeper irritations in the nasal pharynx and can lead to ear infections in children or nose bleeds in older children and adults. If repeated episodes of sinus congestion occur, the cause should be determined by your natural physician. If bacterial infections are present the condition is termed sinusitis, and when it is not properly treated, pneumonia can result. Prescription antibiotics are becoming less effective against these types of infections due to their over use.

TREATMENT: These are techniques I have used in my clinic over the years that are very effective in reducing sinus congestion and sinusitis of all types. Drink 2 to 6 cups of hot *G'Day Melaleuca Tea* each day as a decongestant. Note: For Adults Only. To 1/4 cup of warm *G'Day Melaleuca Tea*, add 1/8 tsp. of table salt. From a cup, snort the mixture into your nose. Tilt your head back and hold it in your sinuses for 10 to 15 seconds. Expel the mixture through your nostrils into a sink. Blow your nose gently. Repeat morning and evening. Dab *T36-C7* directly under each nostril. Breathe the enriched steam from a vaporizer or a bowl of very hot water each morning and night before bed. To do this: Add 5 drops of *T36-C7* to the water or receptacle in front of the steam jet. Form a tent over your head and the vaporizer breathing the aromatic vapors through your nose and mouth deeply and gently into your lungs. Keep your eyes closed. Add 1 or 2 drops of *T36-C7* every 5 minutes for 15 to 20 minutes. Repeat each morning and evening. Apply *Pain-A-Trate* on the temples and forehead to reduce pain from the congestion. Repeat every 2 to 4 hours for relief. If congestion exists, use *CounterAct*, 1 tablet 3-4 times per day.

SNEEZING

Irritations in the nasal pharynx stimulate local histamine production that increases mucous secretion and triggers the central nervous response to expel the irritant. Food or chemical allergies, sensitivities such as hay fever, and viral infections provoke this response. A sneeze is the most efficient way to spread viruses and many bacteria to your family, work mates and friends. The velocity of air and atomized mucous exiting the nose and mouth approaches the speed of sound! Studies show that particles can be projected up to 20 feet across a room from a sneeze. See the section on Air Purification in this book.

TREATMENT: Take *The Vitality Pak* with each meal. Drink 2 to 4 cups of *G'Day Melaleuca Tea* each day. Launder handkerchiefs and rinse in a solution of 1 oz *Sol-U-Mel* per gallon of rinse water. Air dry. For acute sneezing attacks, put 1 or 2 drops of *T36-C7* on a cotton tipped applicator and swab the inside of each nostril. NOTE: A vaporizer/atomizer with *Sol-U-Mel* is not advised, as the surgical grade of green soap can cause irritation to the lungs. If congestion exists, use *CounterAct*, 1 tablet 3-4 times per day.

SORE GUMS

Damage from rough foods, over zealous flossing, or from a tooth brush needs immediate attention to prevent secondary infections and canker sores. Poor dental hygiene or accumulated plaque below the gum line can lead to periodontal infections. See your dentist or dental hygienist without delay. Many health problems stem from improper dental health.

TREATMENT: Following an injury, immediately swish your mouth with *Breath-Away*. Follow the printed directions. Apply *T36-C7* to the sore area with your finger or a cotton swab to reduce the soreness.

SORE THROAT

The challenge to our body's immune system comes partly from the air we breathe, fluids we drink, and the food we eat. Viruses, bacteria, allergens, pollutants, prescription drugs and over using our voice can produce a sore throat. Many people get a sore throat if they do not get enough rest. Whatever the cause, proper treatment is necessary to prevent the condition from escalating. Cancer of the throat starts with a mild chronic sore throat with or without a cough. See the sections on Coughing and Hoarseness in this book. For more information, call *HEALTH TALK* and consult topic 33.

TREATMENT: Gargle with *Breath-Away* Mouthwash to reduce bacteria and viruses. Swab the back of the throat and tonsil area with a cotton tipped swab saturated with *T36-C7*. (This is my son's first recollection of Melaleuca oil.) If the soreness returns or does not diminish, consult your natural physician.

STIFF NECK

Muscle injuries or viral infections occasionally result in chronic muscle tension in the neck or torticollis. There can be an involuntary pulling of the head to one side. Every chiropractor has managed this type of problem using manual manipulation, massage, deep muscle therapy, electro therapy, exercise, and nutrition. See the section on Athletic Injuries in this book. For more information, call *HEALTH TALK* and consult topic 54.

TREATMENT: See your natural physician for specific guidance. Apply *T36-C7* or *Pain-A-Trate* to the affected muscle 3 times each day and one hour before chiropractic care or physical therapy. Drink 2 to 4 cups of *G'Day Melaleuca Tea* each day. Take *The Vitality Pak* with each meal. Keep affected muscles warm. Avoid breezes or too rapid cool-down after exercise.

STINGING NETTLES

An organic acid found in the spines of the mature nettles plant can pack a powerful sting when punctured into the skin. A red, stinging rash results, which becomes quite painful if untreated. (Actually, the young tender plant, when steamed, is a delicious vegetable that we have savored when camping. Eat them before they sting you!)

TREATMENT: Immediately wash with *Antibacterial Liquid Soap*. Apply *T36-C7* or *Pain-A-Trate* approximately once an hour to the affected area. Usually no more than 3 or 4 treatments is needed.

TAPEWORMS

Infected meat from beef, pork, poultry, or fish which is improperly cooked can carry live cysts of the tapeworm. Although the condition is common in Africa, the Middle East, South America, and Mexico, people in North America usually get tapeworms only when raw fish or meat is consumed on a regular basis (Sushi bars). The multi-segmented parasite can grow to be 10 feet long in the lower bowel. The infected person seldom has any obvious symptoms. Symptoms that are occasionally observed are abdominal pain, diarrhea, and weight loss. Occasionally, the person may feel active worms near the anus. Cellophane tape pressed against the anal opening before retiring at night can detect the eggs which can be seen under a microscope. Blood testing for antibodies or eosinophils can often assist in a positive diagnosis. Diagnosis should be made by your natural physician.

TREATMENT: Cooking meat, poultry, or fish to 133 degrees F (56 degrees C) for at least 5 minutes is necessary to kill the cysts. Native Australians have used _G'Day Melaleuca Tea_ and fresh leaf to eradicate tape worms. Taking _The Vitality Pak_ and drinking the _G'Day Melaleuca Tea_ with each meal is a good preventive if food quality is a concern.

TEETHING

Tooth bud swelling and eruption through the gum is often a stressful experience for parents as well as infants. Teething often is accompanied by a runny nose and loose stool in 6 mo. to 2 year olds.

TREATMENT: The cold, mushy consistency of a piece of frozen banana or grape held so the baby can gum it is the quickest way I have found to speed tooth eruption. We have had mothers make _G'Day Melaleuca Tea_ and honey frozen popsicles that give the same results.

TEMPOROMANDIBULAR JOINT DYSFUNCTION

Temporomandibular Joint Dysfunction Syndrome or TMJ for short, is an extremely painful inflammatory condition caused by improper jaw development, improper dental bite, traumatic injury to the face and jaw, or muscle tension in neck and jaw muscles.

Your teeth are capable of biting with 5,000 pounds per square inch of force. The jaw joint in front of your ear must also carry this force. Damage to the TMJ disk is a direct cause of the aggravating pain. If left untreated, complete degeneration of the joint can take place, requiring surgery.

If the TMJ joint itself is not injured, the condition is called myofascial pain-dysfunction (MPD) syndrome. This condition is common and is aggravated by emotionally stressful situations. The individual usually has a history of clenching and grinding their teeth. People with this condition will have tenderness to the touch in one or more of the chewing muscles, limited ability to open the mouth, and clicking or *"popping"* sounds are quite common.

TREATMENT: TMJ syndrome needs professional advice from your natural physician or dentist. Management may require the use of a night guard splint, and therapy by several specialists. In the mean time, apply *Pain-A-Trate* 2 to 3 times per day to the affected muscles around the jaw joint. This is especially effective for MPD syndrome. Get an upper body massage weekly to relieve neck and facial muscle tension. Take *The Vitality Pak* with each meal and drink 2 to 4 cups of *G'Day Melaleuca Tea* each day. Avoid foods that are hard to chew.

THRUSH

Thrush is a fungal infection of the mouth or throat, caused by the *Candida albicans* organism. Oral yeast infections are common in persons who are on drug therapy. The condition causes the tongue, gums, inside of cheeks and throat to have a white patched and swollen appearance. Repeated use of anti-yeast drugs tends to produce resistant strains.

TREATMENT: Use *Breath-Away*, as directed, for a mouthwash every 2 hours. Brush with *Tooth Polish*. Drink 2 to 6 cups of *G'Day Melaleuca Tea* daily. Take *The Vitality Pak* with each meal. For severe infections, dab *T36-C7* on the area or apply with a finger or cotton tipped swab. Avoid sugar and alcohol.

TINNITIS

Unexplained noises such as buzzing, ringing, roaring, whistling, or hissing are heard by sufferers of this condition. It can be in one or both ears. Tinnitis can be a symptom of almost any disorder of or around the ear. It may be caused by low grade infections, anemia, trauma to the head, obstructions such as ear wax, Eustachian tube obstruction from allergies, hardening of the acoustic arteries, tumors, toxicity from chemicals such as carbon monoxide, heavy metal poisoning, many drug reactions, and alcohol. See your natural physician. For more information, call HEALTH TALK and consult topic 26.

TREATMENT: If an organic cause cannot be identified, decongestion is the next best approach. See the section on Chest Congestion in this book. If congestion exists, use CounterAct, 1 tablet 3-4 times per day.

TOBACCO POISONING

The violent effects to the body when tobacco smoke or the masticated juice from smokeless tobacco are consumed testifies to the body's repulsion of such a poison. Animals in nature will not eat the plant. The dried juice from tobacco has been mixed in water to repel garden and household pests and kill plant fungus. In humans, the symptoms of tobacco poisoning include excitement, confusion, muscular twitching, weakness, abdominal cramps, convulsions, depression, rapid respiration, heart palpitations, physical collapse, coma, paralysis and respiratory failure. When levels of nicotine in the blood fall below a certain threshold level, a person with nicotine addiction experiences the same symptoms nicotine poisoning. This level is different for each individual person. In times of excitement, nicotine is degraded and excreted through the kidneys at a faster rate, which causes the addict to crave ingestion even more. Elderly people who have consumed tobacco products for many years show abnormal electrocardiograms, and restricted blood flow to the heart, brain, kidneys, pancreas and extremities.

It is now alleged that the tobacco companies have been *fortifying* cigarette tobacco with extra nicotine, to strengthen its' addictive potential. More than 100 tobacco related deaths occur each day. Hopefully, the public outcry for protection will lead to restrictions on this dangerous substance. Chronic exposure to the substances in tobacco eventually breaks down immune response to infections, and thickens the membranes in the throat and vocal cords. The typical deep raspy voice, dry throat, itching nose and morning coughing fits follow.

TREATMENT: Poisoning from tobacco is linked to at least 50% of the deaths from cancer, heart disease and respiratory

disorders. There is no greater single health measure you can take than to quit smoking and forbid the practice in your home or around your loved ones. Like any drug addiction, it must be faced with courage and compassion. If you have the personal strength to stop smoking - do it right now! If you need help, seek professional care. Have a *Vitality For Life Personal Health Risk Appraisal* performed, and begin a lifestyle of wellness, rather than self destruction. Take *The Vitality Pak* every meal. Take *ProVex* or *ProVex-Plus* daily for antioxidant protection. Drink 2 to 4 cups of *G'Day Melaleuca Tea* each day. Exercise regularly. If congestion exists, use *CounterAct*, 1 tablet 3-4 times per day.

TONSILLITIS

Tonsillitis is an acute inflammation of the tonsillar lymph tissue in the throat, usually due to a Streptococcal bacteria or virus. Epidemics of viral tonsillitis occur in the military or during summer camp. Symptoms in older children and adults include a sore throat upon swallowing and congested Eustachian tubes. Young children will not complain of a sore throat, but will refuse to eat. High fever, headache, and general fatigue are common. The enlarged, and often reddened, tonsils can be seen on either side of the back of the throat. Repeated treatments with antibiotics tend to produce resistant strains of bacteria. See the sections on Air Purification, Disinfectants and Sore Throat in this book. . For more information, call *HEALTH TALK* and consult topics 32 and 33.

TREATMENT: The general health and age of the individual is of the utmost importance in treatment of this condition. For viral tonsillitis, drink *G'Day Melaleuca Tea* every hour. Apply *T36-C7* directly on the tonsils. You may use a cotton tipped swab. Gargle with *Breath-Away* 3 times each day, following the directions for use. A positive culture is needed to confirm bacterial tonsillitis. See your natural physician. Until a definitive diagnosis is made, apply *T36-C7* to the tonsils each hour. Drink *G'Day Melaleuca Tea* and take *The Vitality Pak* with each meal. NOTE:

Improperly treated bacterial tonsillitis can lead to strep throat, rheumatic heart disease and a chronically compromised immune system. Do not self-treat this one. Seek professional help. If congestion exists, use *CounterAct*, 1 tablet 3-4 times per day.

TOOTH ACHE

Dental problems are more easily prevented than treated at home. A sensitive tooth, due to root exposure, thin enamel, or cavities can begin aching from things such as sweets, hot or cold foods, or an uneven bite plane. See the section on Abscesses in this book. For more information, call *HEALTH TALK* and consult topic 30.

TREATMENT: Brush with *Tooth Polish* after every meal. Use *Breath-Away* as a mouthwash after every meal. Use Melaleuca *Dental Tape with T36-C7* at least once each day. Apply *T36-C7* directly to the sensitive tooth and surrounding gum to achieve immediate relief. Have regular checkups with your dentist to maximize the general health of your teeth.

ULCERS

Over stimulation of the Vagus nerve from the brain, too much coffee, rich foods, alcohol, emotional stress, aspirin or drug toxicity can cause esophageal, stomach or duodenum ulcers. Acid in the stomach causes erosion of the mucous lining, resulting in bleeding, anemia and fatigue. One out of every 10 adults develops ulcers at one time or another in their life. About one half of the patients with ulcers experience a pain, gnawing, soreness, hunger, or constant empty feeling. The other half have no symptoms, but show signs of blood in their stool. Our modern *"hurry up"* society seems to produce more people with ulcers than ever before. Our office test for stomach acid production often identifies people developing ulcers before any symptoms occur.

TREATMENT: Have a *Vitality For Life Personal Health Risk Appraisal* performed and begin following the recommendations. **Learn to manage stress more efficiently and take time to enjoy your food. Take *The Vitality Pak* with each meal. Use *This Is Fiber?* as a snack between meals. Drink *G'Day Melaleuca Tea* between meals to revive normal mucous membranes.**

URINARY TRACT INFECTIONS

Almost any normal skin organism is capable of living in the nutrient rich, moist, and dark environment found in the lower urinary tract. Women are more prone to UTI's because of the constant moist environment of the urethral opening and its close proximity to the anus. I have found that fewer than one half of the women with UTI's have any symptoms of the illness. Tight fitting clothes, prescription drug reactions, synthetic undergarments, warm weather, inadequate toilet hygiene, or a generally weakened immune system can lead to bacterial or yeast infections in the urinary tract. Usually, drinking enough water tends to prevent or overcome many of these shortcomings. If improperly treated, UTI's can progress to bladder infections (cystitis) or kidney infection (nephritis).

TREATMENT: The best treatment is prevention. Use cotton panties. Dry your body well after showering or bathing. Drink enough water and 4 to 12 cups of *G'Day Melaleuca Tea* each day. Take *The Vitality Pak* with each meal. Douche as needed during warm weather with *Nature's Cleanse*. If results are not achieved with these suggestions, contact your natural physician for further advice.

VAGINITIS

Bacteria and yeasts can infect the nutrient rich vaginal lining causing painful swelling, foul odor, colored discharge and reduced libido. The increase in sexual promiscuity in the young, and the overuse of antibiotics for every *"ism"* and *"itis"* that comes along has produced super strains of organisms that cause drug defying infections of the female organs. A history of pelvic inflammatory disease is a leading factor in infertility. Reoccurring vaginitis is the most common historical finding. See the sections on Urinary Tract

Infections, Yeast Infections, and Bathing in this book. For more information, call *HEALTH TALK* and consult topics 78, 81, and 83 .

TREATMENT: For acute infections, use *Nature's Cleanse* Feminine Douche morning and evening for 3 to 5 days. For reoccurrences or chronic infections, douche each night. Bathe instead of showering each night, soaking for 30 minutes in a solution of 1 oz of *Sol-U-Mel* and 1 oz of *Natural Spa & Bath Oil*. Avoid sugar. Drinking 2 to 6 cups of *G'Day Melaleuca Tea* each day and 2 to 3 quarts of water per day, along with *The Vitality Pak* with each meal, helps build resistance to infections.

VARICOSE VEINS

Enlarged veins in the lower legs are common among civilized people because of standing and walking on flat hard surfaces all day. Chronic constipation and pregnancy also tend to cause circulation back-up in the legs, which leads to varicose veins. Occasionally there is leg pain or discomfort, but usually not. Valves in veins normally prevent blood from flowing backward or pooling. Sedentary lifestyle destroys this check-valve effect and leads to pooling. Varicose veins and hemorrhoids are often found together. Toe action, like walking barefoot on a sandy beach, assists the pumping of blood back to the heart and keeps leg veins and their check-valves healthy. Using a clinical examination for venous circulation, we often find the beginnings of blood clots blocking this natural flow. Some scientists feel that most blood clots plugging brain (stroke) and heart (heart attack) arteries originate in the oxygen depleted veins of the legs. See the section on Constipation in this book. For more information, call *HEALTH TALK* and consult topic 61.

TREATMENT: We have treated people successfully for varicose veins by following a few simple suggestions. Elderly people may require specialized care beyond these suggestions. Do not wear tight fitting belts or girdles. Wear support hose ONLY when walking or standing for prolonged periods of time. Wearing them while sitting or driving can cause more circulation problems than it helps. Walk barefoot for 10 minutes each morning in the dew or on a sandy beach!

(This is my prescription for Hawaiians.) Maintain healthy regular bowel movements - you should not have to strain at making a stool. Take *ProVex* or *ProVex-Plus* daily to promote vascular integrity. Drink 2 to 6 cups of *G'Day Melaleuca Tea* each day and eat one or two *This Is Fiber?* bars each day for added bowel motility.

WARTS

Common warts, also known as verruca, are non-cancerous tumors caused by pathoviruses. Under microscopic examination, the flat plates of the epidermis are seen to be tilted at ninety degrees, growing outward instead of lying flat with the skin surface. Otherwise, the skin cells appear normal. Viral warts most frequently grow on the hands or fingers of children. The elbows, knees, face, and isolated sites elsewhere on the body are less common. They appear most frequently on sites subject to injury. The appearance and size depends upon the location and on the degree of irritation they are subjected to. They can be round or irregular, and are usually firm and dry. Color varies from light gray, yellow, brown to grayish black. Size varies from 1/8 to 1/2 inch. They may come and go in the same individual in a haphazard way. Infections with the virus may persist as single or multiple growths, and develop by spreading from one side of the body to the other. Complete regression is common, with or without treatment. Warts can persist for years and may reoccur at the same or different sites.

Plantar warts are common on the sole of the foot. When they are flattened by pressure, they are surrounded by cornified tissue and may be very tender. They can be distinguished from corns and calluses by their tendency to pinpoint bleeding when the surface is shaved away.

Filiform warts are long narrow growths usually seen on the eyelids, face, neck or lips. Flat warts are smooth, flat yellow brown lesions seen more commonly in children and young adults, most often on the face. Warts of unusual shape which resemble cauliflower or other structures are most frequent on the head and neck, especially the scalp and in the bearded regions.

Warts around the moist genital area are often called venereal warts and may or may not resemble warts in other parts of the body.

TREATMENT: For isolated common warts, apply *T36-C7* each morning and night faithfully for up to 3 weeks. If the wart is thick and dry, shave the excess away before applying *T36-C7*. For body warts, bathe in a hot tub with 1 oz of *Sol-U-Mel* and 1 oz of *Natural Spa & Bath Oil* for 30 minutes. Apply *T36-C7, Problem Skin Lotion* or *Mela-Gel* afterward. Some warts require the added strength of *T40-C5* to disappear. A few warts do not respond to Melaleuca oil.

YEAST INFECTIONS

Yeasts such as *Candida albicans* can be cultured from the stool of every human. They can be found in the stool of babies only a few days old. Yeasts are actually of the plant kingdom and live only on dead or decaying matter. Spores float in the air freely from decaying matter in the soil of indoor as well as outdoor plants. Yeasts do not tend to activate the body's immune defenses except in overgrowth situations. They are naturally kept from growing out of control by neighboring friendly bacteria which secrete anti-yeast chemicals. These friendly bacteria are innocently destroyed by broad spectrum antibiotics given for other conditions. These friendly bacteria are also inhibited from producing their protective chemicals by taking prescription drugs, hormones, birth control pills, or chemotherapy. When the body is left unprotected by these friendly bacteria, yeast can have a picnic on the nutrient rich protein found on the skin and sugar enriched mucous membranes . Yeast infections are virtually nonexistent in people who eat simple whole foods. Once yeast infections get started, the *"new kid on the block"* must be dealt with in an aggressive, holistic way for best results. Each body site and complicating condition must be addressed on an individual basis for lasting affects. See the sections on Air Purification, Body Odor, Decayed Teeth, Diaper Rash, Emphysema, Jock Itch, Mucous, Paronychia, Thrush, Urinary Tract Infections and Vaginitis in this book for specific details.

TREATMENT: Drink *G'Day Melaleuca Tea* and take *Vitality Pak* with each meal. Avoid sugar, yeast, or mold processed foods. Apply *T36-C7, Mela-Gel, Triple Antibiotic Ointment*, or *Problem Skin Lotion* to the affected areas.

PERSONAL NOTES

PERSONAL NOTES

HEALTHY HOME GUIDE

Being raised with many people coming and going in our home and having a variety of animals to love and play with has taught me a lot. I learned how to clean a cut on a cow or horse at an early age, and how to have a house looking sparkling clean in just the nick of time.

Now, as a wife and mother, I am applying what I was taught to my every day life. My husband, daughter, and I live in the city but still have a *"mini farm"*. As a child care provider, I now have many little finger prints on the windows, crayon marks on the walls, and juice spills on the floor. I have really appreciated using all of the Melaleuca products.

The fact that all the products are environmentally safe as well as non-toxic is an added bonus. Our home is now the First-Aid station in the neighborhood because of our wonderful Melaleuca Oil.

It is a great privilege to share a few of my personal experiences with you as well as working on this book with my father, Dr. Brouse. I wish you good luck in making your home sparkling clean and giving your family and pets optimum health by using quality Melaleuca products.

Julie Brouse-Conrad

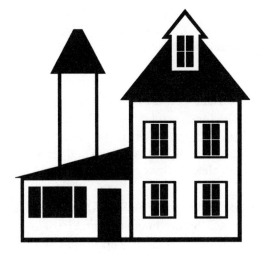

BATHROOM

BATHTUB - Mix 2 Tablespoons *Tub 'N Tile* with 10 ounces of water. Spray on tub and let sit for about 2 minutes. Wipe clean with damp cloth. For rust spots, apply straight *Tub 'N Tile* to area. Wait until rust dissolves then wipe away with a damp cloth. For hard water or mineral deposits, use full strength with a soft scrub brush. Initially there may be strong fumes due to the quantity of build up being dissolved, so run the fan or open a window. This problem should disappear very soon if *Tub 'N Tile* is used on a regular basis.

FLOOR - Mix 2 Tablespoons of *MelaMagic* and 1 cap full of *Sol-U-Mel* with 16 ounces of water. I keep this in a spray bottle, but it can be mixed in a bucket. Spray or wipe on the floor and mop it up.

SINK - Mix 4 Tablespoons of *Tub 'N Tile* and one cap full of *Sol-U-Mel* mixed with 16 ounces of water in a spray bottle. Spray sink and wipe down with damp cloth. For rust stains or mineral deposits, use *Tub 'N Tile* full strength. You may need to use a soft bristle brush on stubborn stains. Rinse clean with water.

SHOWER CURTAIN - Mix 2 Tablespoons of *MelaMagic* & 1 cap full of *Sol-U-Mel* with 10 ounces of water in a spray bottle. Spray on curtain and let sit for a few minutes. Wipe clean with a damp cloth.

TOILET - Pour 4 Tablespoons of *Tub 'N Tile* in toilet, let it sit for a few minutes and then scrub clean with a toilet brush. If you have great build up, turn the water off on your toilet and let it drain. Pour 4 Tablespoons of *Tub 'N Tile* in and let it sit a few minutes and then scrub clean with a brush.

COUNTER - Add one cap full of *Sol-U-Mel* to 10 Ounces of water in a spray bottle. Spray on counter and let it sit a few minutes. Wipe clean with a damp cloth. This will kill any germs that may be on your counter.

MIRROR - I use either the *ClearPower* or a solution of 2 drops of *Tough 'N Tender* in 16 ounces of water. Works great.

CEILINGS - Mix 5 drops of *Tough 'N Tender* with 10 ounces of water in a spray bottle. Apply on ceiling and wipe clean with damp cloth. For real dirty or greasy ceilings, I use 2 Tablespoons of *MelaMagic* with 16 ounces of water in a spray bottle.

WALLS - Mix 5 drops of *Tough 'N Tender* with 10 ounces of water in a spray bottle. Apply on walls and wipe clean with a damp cloth.

TILE - Mix 5 drops of *Tough 'N Tender* with 10 ounces of water in a bucket or a spray bottle. Apply and wipe clean with a damp cloth.

UNDER COUNTERS - Mix 5 drops of *Tough 'N Tender* with 1/2 cap of *Sol-U-Mel* and 16 ounces of water. The addition of *Sol-U-Mel* to the *Tough 'N Tender* mixture, takes care of any mold or mildew problem under the counter.

KITCHEN

MICROWAVE - Mix 5 drops of *Tough 'N Tender* with 16 ounces of water in a spray bottle. Apply and wipe clean with a damp cloth.

STOVE - For minor clean up, use 5 drops of *Tough 'N Tender* with 16 ounces of water in a spray bottle. Apply and let it sit for a few minutes and then wipe clean with a cloth. For major clean up apply *MelaMagic* full strength with a cloth. Let it sit for a few minutes and then use a soft scrubbing pad to lift off grime. Wipe clean with a damp cloth.

STOVE HOOD (ventilation hood) - Use *MelaMagic* full strength on a cloth. Apply and let sit a few minutes and then wipe clean with a damp cloth.

OVEN - Use 4 Tablespoons *MelaMagic* and 1 cap full of *Sol-U-Mel* with 16 ounces of water in a spray bottle. Apply and let sit for 5 minutes and then wipe clean with a damp cloth. If it is a major job, use a soft scrubbing pad and straight *MelaMagic*.

STOVE TOP RINGS - Mix 4 Tablespoons of *MelaMagic* in a bucket or sink full of water. Put rings in and let them soak for 5 minutes, wipe clean and rinse off with water.

COUNTERS - Mix 5 drops of *Tough 'N Tender* with 16 ounces of water in a spray bottle. Spray on counters and wipe clean with cloth. For removing stubborn stains, sprinkle a little *Diamond Brite* on the stain. Wipe it off with a damp cloth.

SINK - For general cleaning, put a few drops of *Tough 'N Tender* into the sink and scrub clean with a soft brush. To whiten or shine a sink, I sprinkle a little bit of *Diamond Brite* on the sink and then scrub it clean. Watch it sparkle!!

TOASTER OVEN - Use either the *ClearPower* solution or 5 drops of *Tough 'N Tender* with 16 ounces of water in a spray bottle. Spray on toaster oven and wipe clean with a cloth.

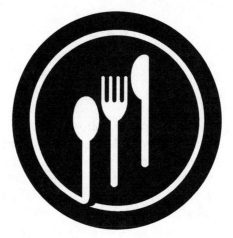

TELEPHONE - Mix 5 drops of *Tough 'N Tender* with 1/2 cap of *Sol-U-Mel* in 16 ounces of water. Spray on phone and wipe off with cloth.

TILE - Mix 5 drops of *Tough 'N Tender* with 16 ounces of water. Spray on and wipe off.

FRUIT & VEGETABLES - Place fruit or vegetables in a bowl of water containing 1 drop of *Tough 'N Tender*. Let fruit or vegetables sit for about 5 minutes and then rinse clean. This will remove dirt, sprays, or wax from the fruit or vegetables.

WINDOWS - Spray with *ClearPower* or a mixture of water and 5 drops of *Tough 'N Tender*.

FLOORS - Mix 1 Tablespoon of *MelaMagic* with a bucket full of hot water. Mop the floor and let air dry.

REFRIGERATOR - Mix 5 drops of *Tough 'N Tender* with 1/2 cap of *Sol-U-Mel* and add to 16 ounces of water in a spray bottle. Spray the inside and outside of fridge with this solution and wipe dry with cloth.

CUPBOARD - To clean the outside of the cupboard, mix 1 Tablespoon of *MelaMagic* with 16 ounces of water. Spray cupboard and wipe clean with cloth. For the inside of cupboard, add 5 drops of *Tough 'N Tender* to 16 ounces of water. Spray and wipe clean.

DISHWASHER - To clean the outside of the dishwasher, use 5 drops of *Tough 'N Tender* with 16 ounces of water. Spray on and wipe clean with a cloth. Only use 1 tablespoon of *Diamond Brite* in your dishwasher to clean dishes. If you have hard or soft water, this measurement may need to be adjusted.

FREEZER - To clean spills, use 5 drops of *Tough 'N Tender* with 16 ounces of water. Spray on and wipe clean with a cloth. To kill mold or mildew, use 1 cap full of *Sol-U-Mel* with 16 ounces of water. Spray on and let sit for 5 minutes. Wipe clean with a cloth.

HAND DISHES - Use 5 to 7 drops of *MelaDrops* in a sink full of water. For baked on food fill container with hot water to which 2 to 3 drops of *MelaDrops* have been added. Let soak for 1/2 hour and then wipe clean.

STAINS - Soak stained dishes or china in a bucket or sink of hot water containing 1/3 cup of *Diamond Brite*. Let soak for 1 hour. If stain has not dissolved, soak it over night.

CEILING/WALLS - Mix 4 Tablespoons of *MelaMagic* in a bucket of hot water. Use cloth to wash down ceiling or walls with solution. Let air dry.

BRASS - Mix 2 Tablespoons of *Tub 'N Tile* with 16 ounces of water. Spray on brass piece and wipe off with clean cloth.

COPPER - Mix 2 ounces of *Tub 'N Tile* with 16 ounces of water. Spray on copper pieces and wipe off with a clean cloth.

LIVING ROOM

CARPET DEODORIZATION - Mix 1 cap full of *Sol-U-Mel* in 10 ounces of water. Spray on carpet and let it sit for 5 minutes. Clean with a scrub brush. Blot with a damp cloth until clean.

CARPET SPOT CLEANING - Mix 2 Tablespoons of *Pre-Spot* with 1/2 cap full of *Sol-U-Mel* and 16 ounces of water in a spray bottle. Apply solution to soiled area. Let sit for 5 minutes and then clean with a soft brush. Blot with a damp cloth until clean.

COMPLETE CARPET CLEANING - Mix 1/4 cup of *Pre-Spot*, 1/2 Cup of *MelaMagic*, and 1 tablespoon of *Sol-U-Mel*. Pour solution into the tray of the carpet cleaner. This works wonderfully! (First test this on a small area of carpet for color fastness.)

WOOD FLOORS - Mix 5 drops of *Tough 'N Tender* with 16 ounces of water. Spray on floor and then wipe dry with cloth.

GLASS - Apply *ClearPower* to glass and then wipe dry with a cloth or paper towel.

DUSTING - Mix 5 drops of *Tough 'N Tender* with 16 ounces of water. Spray on a cloth and wipe onto dusty area.

FURNITURE - For spot cleaning, use 2 Tablespoons *Pre-Spot* with 16 ounces of water. You may want to test it first on a hidden area.

GLASS TABLE TOPS - Apply 1/2 teaspoon *MelaSoft* and 1 quart water. Spray or wipe on. Dry with cloth towel. This will keep lint off.

FIREPLACE - For the fire place glass, use *ClearPower*. For the outside of the fire place, use 2 Tablespoons of *MelaMagic* with 16 ounces of water. Spray on soiled area and scrub clean.

WALLS/CEILING - Mix 5 drops of *MelaMagic* with 16 ounces of water. Apply by either spraying on or wiping on with a cloth.

CRAYON/MARKER MARK - Mix 5 drops of *Tough 'N Tender* with 16 ounces of water. If you need more cleaning strength, use 1 Tablespoon of *MelaMagic* with 1/2 cap of *Sol-U-Mel*. Scrub clean.

BLINDS - Mix 5 drops of *Tough 'N Tender* with 1/2 cap *Sol-U-Mel* and 16 ounces of water. Close blinds, spray on solution and wipe dry with a cloth.

CEILING FAN - Mix 5 drops of *Tough 'N Tender* with 16 ounces of water. Spray on fan and wipe off with a cloth.

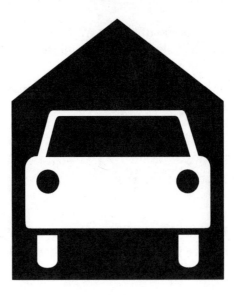

GARAGE

GREASE SPILLS - Pour full strength *MelaMagic* on grease spot and let it sit for 15 minutes; then wipe clean.

GAS SPILLS - Soak a cloth with *MelaMagic*. Wipe up spill. You may also try adding some *Sol-U-Mel* on the cloth as well.

CAR CLEANING - For dusting the inside, spray a solution of 5 drops of *Tough 'N Tender* with 16 ounces of water on a cloth. Wipe clean. For windows, spray on *ClearPower* and wipe clean. For cleaning the outside of the car, fill a bucket with warm water and 10 drops of *Tough 'N Tender*. Apply with cloth and spray off with clean water.

MACHINE PARTS - Mix 2 Tablespoons of *MelaMagic* and 16 ounces of water. Spray on part and let sit. Wipe clean with damp cloth. If the part is grimy, soak the part in the above solution, then scrape off as much of the build up as possible. Remove the remainder with a stiff brush (natural, wire or brass) kept wet with the cleaning solution. For small parts, soak a rag in either full strength *MelaMagic* or in the solution and wipe the part clean.

GREASY HANDS - Using the *Gold Bar* works well or try a little bit of *MelaMagic*. Rub hands together and then rinse with water.

GARBAGE CAN - Pour 1/4 cup of *MelaMagic* and 1 cap full of *Sol-U-Mel* into garbage can. Fill can 1/4 full of hot water and then scrub sides with a soft brush. Pour mixture out and rinse clean with water.

TAR - Soak a cloth with *Sol-U-Mel* and wipe effected area. This should dissolve the tar right away.

SAW BLADES - To clean resin build-up from saw blades, shaper bits, or router bits, apply *MelaMagic* full strength. Wipe clean with a damp cloth. Soaking or scrubbing with a soft bristled brush may be necessary. Dry thoroughly and coat with a thin film of light oil (3-in-1, WD 40, vegetable oil, etc.) to guard against rusting.

LAUNDRY ROOM

WASHER - Before running your first load of wash using *MelaPower* laundry detergent, it is best to run the washer empty with just 1/4 cup *MelaPower* laundry detergent to clean all the lines. After you have done that, run a load of wash using 1/8 cup *MelaPower* laundry detergent. To whiten your laundry load, add either 1 cap full of *Sol-U-Mel* or 2 Tablespoons of *Diamond Brite*. The *Sol-U-Mel* will also deodorize the article of fabric.

BLOOD SPOTS - Spray clothing with full strength *Pre-Spot*. Let sit for a few minutes. Rub it clean under cold water and launder with *MelaPower* laundry detergent.

FRUIT JUICE SPOTS - Spray area with full strength *Pre-Spot*. Let sit a few minutes, then laundry with *MelaPower* launder detergent.

GUM - Pour full strength *Sol-U-Mel* on effected area. Let sit a minute. Rub to loosen up the gum then wash in *MelaPower* laundry detergent.

DIRT - Spray effected area with full strength *Pre-Spot*. Let sit for a few minutes then launder in *MelaPower* laundry detergent.

PET ODOR - Launder fabric in *MelaPower* laundry detergent and a cap full of *Sol-U-Mel*.

CRAYON - Spray effected area with full strength *Pre-Spot*. Let it sit a few minutes, then scrub to loosen crayon from fabric. Wash fabric with *MelaPower* laundry detergent.

FINE WASHABLES - To launder wool, nylon, or other fine fabrics; dissolve 1 teaspoon of *Tough 'N Tender* in a basin of cold water. Hand wash, and rinse in warm water.

GRASS STAINS - Spray *Pre-Spot* on stain. Let sit for a few minutes. Soak soiled clothing in a bucket of warm water containing 2 tablespoons of *MelaPower* laundry detergent for a few hours. Wash as normal.

GREASE SPOTS - Mix a solution of 2 Tablespoons of *MelaPower* laundry detergent and 1 capful of *Sol-U-Mel* with 2 gallons of warm water. Put clothing in bucket of water and let soak for a few hours. If the grease spots are not dissolved, apply a squirt of liquid soap. Rub in with your finger or a soft brush. Let stand for a few minutes before rinsing with warm water.

INK STAINS - Spray *Pre-Spot* on stain and rub with your finger or a soft brush. Let sit for a few minutes and rinse clean in warm water.

LIP STICK STAINS - Spray *Pre-Spot* on stain. Let sit for a few minutes. Soak clothing for a few hours in a 2 gallon bucket of cold water containing 2 Tablespoons of *MelaPower* laundry detergent; then rinse clean with cool water.

PAINT - Spray *Pre-Spot* on paint spot or splatter. Rub with your finger or a soft brush. Let it sit for a few minutes and then rinse in warm water. This method works very well, but some paint stains are there to stay.

CANDLE WAX STAINS - To remove stains from linen or carpeting, press a *warm* iron over a paper towel on the spot. Continue to iron until the wax melts and is absorbed in the paper towel. Then clean area with 1/2 teaspoon *Tough 'N Tender* and 16 ounces of water.

TOYS - Washables - Place all washable, stuffed animals, dollies, and blankies in washing machine. Add 1/8 cup of *MelaPower* laundry detergent and 1 capful of *Sol-U-Mel*. Wash as usual.

BLEACH SUBSTITUTE - Add 1 Tablespoon of *Diamond Brite* to your load of light laundry after the tub has been filled with water on the first cycle.

TREE PITCH - Spray affected areas with *Orchard Mist* hair spray. Let sit for about one minute. Wash clean with *Melaleuca Antibacterial Liquid Soap* and water.

FABRIC DYE STAINS - Spray affected areas with *Pre-Spot*. Let sit for about one minute, then soak in a container with 1/8 cup *MelaPower* for 30 minutes. If the stain is not completely gone, reapply *Pre-Spot* and wash in washing machine with 1/8 cup *MelaPower*. My friend had just washed a load of clothing, and discovered that load contained her beautiful new red blouse along with her husband's new navy blue shirt. The blouse and shirt met in the wash cycle and exchanged colors. I received a frantic call asking me to *"Perform a miracle with my Melaleuca stuff!"* We used the above procedure on both articles and knocked her socks off!

OUTDOOR

CLEANING EXTERIOR OF HOUSE - Mix 2 Tablespoons of *MelaMagic* with 16 ounces of water. Apply solution by either spraying or wiping on. Scrub clean with brush. Rinse with water.

GREASE - Mix 2 parts *MelaMagic* to 8 parts water, or apply straight *MelaMagic* on grease spot. Use a brush to scrub clean. Rinse off with water.

PLANTS - Add 1 Tablespoon of *Tough 'N Tender* to 16 ounces of water. Spray on roses to kill aphids.

BAR-B-QUE - Soak Bar-B-Que grill in a solution of 2 Tablespoons of *MelaMagic* in 1/2 gallon water. Scrub clean with brush. For the outside of the Bar-B-Que, use 1 Tablespoon of *Tough 'N Tender* and 16 ounces of water, spray on Bar-B-Que and scrub clean with a soft brush.

LAWN FURNITURE - Mix 1 teaspoon of *Tough 'N Tender* with 16 ounces of water. Spray on furniture and wipe clean with a cloth.

ALUMINUM, STEEL, AND WROUGHT IRON FURNITURE - Mix 1 Tablespoon of *Tough 'N Tender* with 1 gallon of water. Wash furniture down with a rag or sponge. Rinse clean and dry thoroughly. Once a season, apply a coat of automobile wax (If a scratch occurs on wrought iron or steel, apply machine exterior paint with a small artist brush).

WOOD FURNITURE - To clean dirt from wood furniture, mix 1 teaspoon of *Tough 'N Tender* and 1 gallon of water. Apply with a rag or sponge. Towel dry. For heavy stains, use 1 Tablespoon of *Sol-U-Mel* and 1 gallon of water.

AWNINGS - Add 1 Tablespoon of *Tough 'N Tender* to 1/2 gallon of warm water. Wet a clean cloth with solution. Wipe awning with cloth until clean and then spray off with water.

CONCRETE FLOORS - For general cleaning, use 2 Tablespoons of *MelaMagic* in 1/2 gallon of warm water. Dump a small puddle of solution on floor, and scrub clean. Spray clean with water hose.

LAWN MOWER - To remove dirt and grease marks, mix a solution of 1 Tablespoon of *MelaMagic* with 1/2 gallon of warm water. Use a cloth or rag to scrub clean.

INSECT REPELLENT - For humans mix 1 teaspoon of *Body Satin Lotion* and 5 drops *T36-C7*. Apply to exposed skin. For outside air, mix 2 Tablespoons of *Sol-U-Mel* and 16 ounces of water. Spray into the air around where people are.

WINDOW/DOOR SCREENS - Mix 1 Tablespoon *Tough 'N Tender* with 1 gallon warm water. Dip screen into solution, and scrub clean with a soft brush.

CLAY FLOWER POTS - To clean moss or algae, spray pot with 1 teaspoon *Sol-U-Mel* in 16 ounces of water. Scrub with a stiff brush or steel wool. Rinse clean with water. Towel dry.

HOME/CAR FIRST AID KIT - *T36-C7, Problem Skin Lotion, Triple Antibiotic Ointment, Mela-Gel, Sun-Shades All weather lotion*, scissors, tweezers, Band-Aids, gauze, and a very small container of water (for washing wound).

PET CARE

The hair and skin of most animals should not be overly washed with harsh detergents or shampoos. Cats and dogs can develop a sensitivity and produce dry skin as a result of over washing. However, preventive care during seasonal infestation with fleas, ticks, mites and other insects can be accomplished by proper nutritional support to the animal. Dogs appear to have a particularly high requirement for extra calcium and magnesium. Cats appear to require additional B-Complex, often in the form of Brewers yeast. Both dogs and cats appear to fare very well when treated with *Sol-U-Mel, Natural Spa & Bath Oil*, and *T36-C7*. Optimum nutritional support should be provided based on the individual animal. Your natural veterinarian should be consulted if you are uncertain as to what your pet may need.

FLEA PROTECTION - Wash all bedding in washing machine with 2 caps full of *Sol-U-Mel* and 1/8 cup of *MelaPower* laundry detergent. Add 2 Tablespoons of *Sol-U-Mel* to 16 ounces of water, and apply to areas where your dog or cat sleep or rest during the day and evening. Wash your dog and/or cat with the *ProCare* shampoo. If the fleas are severe add a cap full of *Sol-U-Mel* to the bath water.

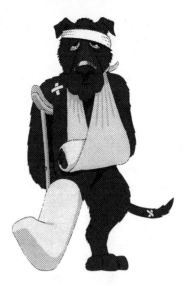

DOGS - Use the *ProCare* animal cleaning products for a healthy, beautiful looking coat. Give *Nutritional Treats* for Dogs every day to enhance their health and give them vim and vigor. These can also be used as a reward in training your dog.

"Hot Spots" and abrasions on the body respond well to *T36-C7* applied frequently to reduce pain, prevent infection and promote healing. *Mela-Gel* can be applied if drying or scaling results. Paw abrasions are treated with *Mela-Gel* or *Triple Antibiotic Ointment*.

For beautiful, shiny coat on dogs shampoo with *ProCare Professional Pet Shampoo*. You will find your pet's coat dries quickly to a shiny luster.

CATS - Ringworm, which is a fungus, can be treated with *T36-C7* very effectively. Be mindful of any signs of sensitivity. Some breeds react to the pure oil in which case *Mela-Gel* or *Triple Antibiotic Ointment* is effective. Bathing the cat in *Sol-U-Mel* 1/2 teaspoon per quart of water is often helpful.

Cat fight scratches heal nicely with *Mela-Gel* after bathing with *Antibacterial Liquid Soap* or *ProCare Professional Pet Shampoo*. Keep in mind that cat scratches are very serious to humans as many disease causing germs are found on cat claws.

150

HORSES - Use *Herbal Shampoo* to wash your horses coat. The *Herbal Shampoo* has a conditioner in it so it will make it easy to get tangles out of the mane and tail.

To control flies in the stall area, mix 1 cap of *Tough 'N Tender* with 16 ounces of water in spray bottle. Apply liberally early in the day. Solution may be sprayed on horses body to repel flies. Cover horses eyes.

For cuts apply a mixture of 2 caps *Natural Spa & Bath Oil*, 3 caps *Sol-U-Mel*, 2 caps *Nature's Cleanse*, 5 drops of *Antibacterial Liquid Soap* in 1 quart of water. Spray several times per day to affected area.

For nail puncture wounds. WARNING! If the nail is still in horses foot, do not remove until a veterinarian has decided to X-ray. The position of the nail near the bone must be determined to predict the outcome of this injury. Horses have very poor circulation in the frog of their feet. Sometimes surgery may be needed! Otherwise, begin soaking the foot in a mixture of 2 caps *Sol-U-Mel*, 1 cap *Antibacterial Liquid Soap* in 2 quarts of warm water for 30 minutes morning and evening. After soaking, apply *T36-C7*, then *Mela-Gel*, and cover with gauze. Repeat for 3 weeks even if horse walks without a limp before this time.

RABBITS - For ear mites, clean ears with Q-tip and then squeeze a dab of *Problem Skin Lotion* on a clean Q-tip and apply to the inside of the ear. Massage ear gently to distribute the lotion evenly. To clean a cage mix 2 Tablespoons *Sol-U-Mel* with 16 ounces of water. Spray on cage and on the bottom tray to clean and deodorize. Scrub clean with a brush. Rinse with water.

HAMSTERS, GERBILS, GUINEA PIGS OR RATS - To control odor in or around a small animal's cage or to prevent communicable diseases, dab *T36-C7* or spray a 1:20 diluted solution of *Sol-U-Mel* to the area 2 or 3 times each week.

PARAKEETS, CANARIES OR TROPICAL BIRDS - To prevent diseases among birds, use a 1:100 dilution of *Sol-U-Mel* sprayed once per week to the absorbent fodder material on the bottom of the cage. Spray each time the fodder is changed. WARNING! Some exotic birds are sensitive to the aromatic oils in *T36-C7*.

SORES - Apply *Problem Skin Lotion* with a drop of *T36-C7* to open wounds . For scrapes apply *Mela-Gel* or *Triple Antibiotic Ointment*.

CLEANING BEDDING - Wash all bedding in the washing machine with 1 cap full of *Sol-U-Mel* and 1/8 cup of *MelaPower* laundry detergent. This will clean as well as deodorize.

CLEANING FEEDING BOWLS - Place 1 drop of *Tough 'N Tender* in each bowl; fill with hot water and scrub clean.

LIVESTOCK (Fly repellent) - Mix 2 Tablespoons of *Sol-U-Mel* with 16 ounces of water. Spray directly on the horse or cow.

ANIMAL FIRST AID KIT - For our outings with horses, we always carry *T36-C7, Triple Antibiotic Ointment, Sol-U-Mel, Mela-Gel,* and *Problem Skin Lotion,* gauze, tape, tweezers, scissors, and water (in a small container for cleaning).

PERSONAL NOTES

PERSONAL NOTES

BIBLIOGRAPHY

Belaiche, P. *Treatment of Skin Infections with The Essential Oil of Melaleuca alternifolia.*: **Phylotherapie** Vol 15, 1985.

Belaiche, P. *Treatment of Vaginal Infections of Candida Albicans with the Essential Oil of Melaleuca alternifolia.* **Phylotherapie** Vol 15, 1985.

Beylier, M.F. *Bacteriostatic activity of some Australian essential oils.* **Perfumes and Flavorings.** 23-5, 4 (2) 1979.

Blackwell, A.L. *Tea Tree Oil and Anaerobic (Bacterial) Vaginosis.* **The Lancet** 337-300 (1991).

Blamann, A. and Melrose, G.J.H. *4-Terpinenol.* **Perfumery Essential Oil Record.** 50, 769 (1959).

Essential Oils - Oil of Melaleuca, Terpinen-4-ol Type. Standards Association of Australia. Standards House, 80 Arthur St. North Sydney, N.S.W. 1985.

Laakso, P.V. *Fractionation of Tea Tree Oil.* **25th Congress of Pharmaceutical Science**, Prague. 1,485-492, 1965.

Maruzzella, J. and Ligouri, L. *The in vitro antifungal activity of essential oils.* **Journal of the American Pharmaceutical Association.** 47,250-4 (1958).

McCulloch, R.N. and Waterhouse, D.F. *Laboratory and field tests of mosquito repellents.* **Australia Council of Science and Industry Research Bulletin.** 213,9-26 (1947).

Murray, K.E. *The essential oils of five western Australian plants.* **Royal Australian Chemical Institute Journal and Proceedings.** 17,398-402 (1950).

Penfold, A.R. and Morrison, F.R. *Australian essential oils in insecticide and repellents.* **Soap, Perfumery and Cosmetics.** 25,933-4 (1952).

Penfold, A.R. *Essential oil of Melaleuca alternifolia.* **Perfumery Essential Oil Record.** 25,121 (1934).

Swords, G. and Hunter, G.L.K. *Composition of Australian Tea Tree Oil (Melaleuca alternifolia).* **Journal of Agricultural Food Chemistry.** 26 (3), 734-737, 1978.

Van Hulssen, C.J. and Meyer, T.M. *Ethereal oils from Melaleuca alternifolia and Melaleuca bracteata.* **Inorganic Nederland-Indie.** 8, VII, 84-7 (1941).

Walker, M. *Clinical Investigation of Australian Melaleuca alternifolia Oil for a Variety of Common Foot Problems.* **Current Podiatry** April, 1972.

Appendix 1

Health Talk, Dr. Brouse's 24 hour health advisor

Do you have a question regarding a health problem discussed in this book? Call *HEALTH TALK*, Dr. Brouse's 24 hour health advisor! This unique *FREE* health advisor was developed and tested on thousands of clinic patients over the last 10 years. It offers, in the convenience and privacy of your home, information that will help you decide if your health concern warrants a visit to your doctor, or if it can be managed at home. It is always on call and able to respond to your concern with the advice you need for optimum health. You get individual attention with specific recommendations for your problem. Because the service is popular, you may encounter an occasional busy signal.

How does it work? First, you must have a touch tone telephone to call *HEALTH TALK* (rotary dial phones do not produce the tones needed to answer the questions). When a particular section of this book directs you to call *HEALTH TALK*, note that topic number. Then call *(503) 654-0538*. The first voice you hear will be Dr. Brouse, welcoming you to *HEALTH TALK*. You will be asked to enter the topic number you are interested in. Using the touch tone buttons on your phone, enter the topic number.

Then *HEALTH TALK* will ask you a series of Yes/No questions. When your answer is *YES*, press the number 1 button on your phone. When your answer is *NO*, press the number 9 button on your phone. Your answer to each question determines what the next question will be. Finally when *HEALTH TALK* has enough information to understand your condition, it will give you specific advice for that particular problem.

Each *HEALTH TALK* profile is unique to your symptom characteristics. It does not duplicate the information in this book. Rather, it is a supplement to this book and helps you determine if your problem can be managed at home, or if you need professional help. If *HEALTH TALK* cannot determine exactly what the problem is, it will advise you to contact Dr. Brouse or the appropriate type of local health professional.

NOTE: Dr. Brouse provides *HEALTH TALK* as a public service and assumes no responsibility for the actions or non-actions

taken by users of the system. If *HEALTH TALK* directs you to consult Dr. Brouse regarding your problem, call (503) 654-3225 during regular business hours to schedule an appointment. If you need to order an educational video tape or more copies of this book, call our toll-free order line (800) 845-2025.

APPENDIX 2

Disinfectant Properties of T36-C7
Compared to Other Agents

The following table is the result of our clinical research and is based upon direct contact of the agent with the organism. Standard concentrations were used. This confirms many other studies regarding the disinfectant ability of *Melaleuca alternifolia* oil which contains at least 37% terpenols and less than 7% cineol. Please note that although many organisms show sensitivity to certain agents, mutant strains are developing which resist control. Many disinfectants are toxic or cause damage to skin when used over a prolonged time period. For these reasons, a number of these agents are no longer used clinically.

Organism

Disinfectant Agent	Staph Aureus	E. Coli	Bacteria Spores	Fungi	Viruses	Candida Albicans
Isopropyl alcohol	sensitive	sensitive	resistant	partial	partial	resistant
Phenolics	sensitive	sensitive	resistant	partial	resistant	partial
Chlorine Solution	sensitive	sensitive	resistant	partial	partial	partial
Iodine Tincture	sensitive	sensitive	resistant	partial	resistant	partial
Acetal-dehyde	sensitive	sensitive	partial	sensitive	sensitive	sensitive
Mercury Salts	sensitive	partial	sensitive	sensitive	sensitive	sensitive
Hexa-chlorophen	sensitive	partial	resistant	sensitive	resistant	resistant
Quaternary Ammonium	sensitive	partial	resistant	partial	resistant	resistant
Boric Acid	partial	partial	resistant	resistant	resistant	resistant
Cidex	sensitive	sensitive	partial	sensitive	sensitive	sensitive
T36-C7	sensitive	sensitive	sensitive	sensitive	sensitive	sensitive

Sensitive	=	Disinfectant agent kills organism
Partial	=	Disinfectant agent is partially effective
Resistant	=	Disinfectant agent does not kill organism

APPENDIX 3

Technical Product Information

Although there are over 300 known species of tea trees (*Melaleuca*) in Australia, only one, the *Melaleuca alternifolia*, is known to have substantial therapeutic properties. The most closely related species to *Melaleuca alternifolia* is the *M. linarifolia* that yields an oil that is somewhat bacteriostatic, but is too high in Cineole, a natural skin irritant.

The pure oil of *Melaleuca alternifolia* is known to contain at least 48 compounds. A few of these compounds are not yet identified. A unique compound, viridiflorene, is found only to exist in Oil of *Melaleuca*. Two other compounds: Terpinen-4-ol and Cineole, are regulated by the Australian Standards Association to designate therapeutic quality.

In Australia, the minimum amount of Terpinen-4-ol allowed is 30%, and the maximum amount of Cineole is 15%. Terpinen-4-ol is one of the more important therapeutic ingredients in the oil. Therefore, one would want oil high in Terpinen-4-ol. And since Cineole is caustic to the skin, the higher quality oil is low in Cineole. High quality oil should have at least 35% Terpinen-4-ol and less than 10% Cineole.

Since pure Oil of *Melaleuca* is entirely natural and the genetics of one tree varies slightly from the other, the quality of oil from one grove of trees may vary substantially from another. In fact, much of the oil that has been distilled from *Melaleuca alternifolia* trees does not meet the minimum standards of quality oil.

Much research still needs to be done to determine exactly why *Melaleuca* oil works as it does and what the exact proportion of each of the 48 compounds produces the most effective blend of oil.

Since there are currently no laws in the United States that define Tea Tree Oil or Oil of *Melaleuca*, it is feasible that a person or company could legally sell products labeled as pure Tea Tree Oil or even pure oil of *Melaleuca alternifolia* that is not oil of *Melaleuca* at all. In fact, several companies have recently begun marketing a synthetic oil which they label as pure Tea Tree Oil, or pure oil of *Melaleuca alternifolia* that does not come from that specific tree at all, but is a blend of other oils containing Terpinen-4-ol and Cineole. In Australia, this would be illegal, but in the United States there are no laws at this time preventing it. We strongly recommend that anyone purchasing products labeled as Oil of *Melaleuca* do so from a reputable firm that has its source of oil and quality of oil well documented.

The 48 known compounds of pure
Melaleuca alternifolia oil

1. α-Pinene
2. Camphene
3. β-Pinene
4. Sabinene
5. Myrcene
6. α-Phellandrene
7. 1,4-Cineole
8. α-Terpinene
9. Limonene
10. 1,8-Cineole
11. γ-Terpinene
12. p-Cymene
13. Terpinolene
14. Hexanol
15. Allyl hexanoate
16. p,α-Dimethyl-styrene
17. (a Sesquiterpene)
18. α-Cubebene
19. (a Sesquiterpene)
20. α-Copaene
21. Camphor
22. α-Gurjunene
23. Linalool
24. (a Sesquiterpene)
25. (unidentified)
26. 1-Terpineol
27. 1-Terpinene-4-ol
28. β-Elemene
29. Caryophyllene
30. (a Sesquiterpene)
31. Aromadendrene
32. β-Terpineol
33. Alloromadendrene
34. (unidentified)
35. Humulene
36. (unidentified)
37. γ-Muurolene
38 α-Terpineol
39. Viridiflorene
40. Piperitone
41. α-Muurolene
42. Piperitol
43. (unidentified)
44. σ-Cadinene
45. 4,10-Dimethyl-7-isopropyl bicyclo [4,4,0]-1,4-decadiene
46. Nerol
47. 8-p-Cymenol
48. Clamenene

APPENDIX 4

Dr. Brouse's Video and Audio Tapes

Produced before live audiences, each presentation is unique in the most current information and practical advice for making health decisions. These tapes give the preventive-minded person the information they need to take charge of their own health. When you know your health options, you can choose your health future, instead of taking the chance of developing disease. Share with a friend and enlighten their thinking. Some of the video tapes are also available on audio. For a free catalog of the titles and program synopsis call (800) 845-2025. A few of the titles available are:

Acne	Hyperactivity
Alcoholism	Hypertension
Allergies	Hypoglycemia
Anemia	Immune system
Arthritis	Kidneys
Back pain	Liver and gall bladder
Cancer	Malabsorption
Candida yeast	Menopause
Circulation	Metabolic exhaustion
Colitis	Multiple sclerosis
Colon health	Osteoporosis
Crohn's disease	Potassium and health
Depression	Premenstrual syndrome
Detoxification	Prostate
Diabetes	Relaxation
Digestion	Skin care
Fatigue	Stress
Glaucoma	Tension Control
Headaches	Viral infections
Healthy hearts	Vitamin C
Hemorrhoids	Women's health

PERSONAL NOTES

INDEX

V

Vaginitis, 131
Varicose Veins, 132
Vertigo - see Dizziness
Vomiting - see Nausea

W

Walls, 139
Walls/Ceiling, 143
Warts, 133

Washer, 145
Water Retention - see Edema
Window/Door Screens, 149
Windows, 141
Wood Floors, 142
Wood Furniture, 148
Wrist Pain - see Carpal Tunnel
    Syndrome

Y

Yeast Infections, 134

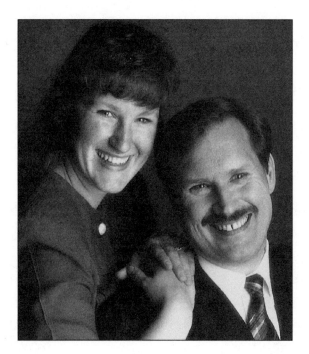

Dr. Richard Brouse received his Masters Degree in Biochemistry from Western States College of Colorado in 1970 and his Doctor of Chiropractic degree from Western States Chiropractic College in Portland, Oregon in 1977. He taught organic chemistry, biochemistry and nutrition at Western States Chiropractic College where he served as Associate Professor of Clinical Nutrition for 14 years.

Dr. Brouse is a widely recognized authority in the fields of nutrition and prevention of chronic degenerative diseases. He is a gifted speaker with the ability to communicate nutritional information in a manner that the general public can understand and personally apply. He has formulated and researched clinical use of *Melaleuca* oil products in his holistic practice.

Julie Brouse-Conrad, the daughter of Dr. Brouse, has grown up in a home that is health and environmentally conscious. She is now a mother and homemaker herself, and enjoys sharing safe ways to care for her home, family, and pets.

NEW RELEASE! - **NOW AVAILABLE:**

Melaleuca Quick Reference

Price for one booklet without shipping: $3.95

The following are the prices per booklet
(including shipping and handling)

Quantity	Continental US	Canada (US Funds) Alaska/Hawaii
1-9	$4.95	$4.95
10-49	$4.05	$4.45
50-99	$3.35	$3.70
100-499	$2.85	$3.20
500-999	$2.40	$2.80
1000-4999	$2.15	$2.40
5000+	$1.95	$2.20

Mail order to:

Health Education Corporation
8800 SE Sunnyside Road, Suite 111
Clackamas, OR 97015

For Telephone Orders with VISA / MasterCard call:
(503) 243-1213 or (800) 845-2025
FAX (503) 654-3056

Name _____ Telephone (____) _____
Street _____
City _____ State ____ Zip Code _____

Number of Books: _____ ○ Check
Amount enclosed: _____ ○ Money Order